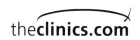

Agnes E. Rupley, DVM, Dipl. ABVP–Avian
CONSULTING EDITOR

VETERINARY CLINICS

OF NORTH AMERICA

Exotic Animal Practice

Renal Disease

GUEST EDITOR
M. Scott Echols, DVM, Dipl. ABVP–Avian

January 2006 • Volume 9 • Number 1

SAUNDERS

An Imprint of Elsevier, Inc.
PHILADELPHIA   LONDON   TORONTO   MONTREAL   SYDNEY   TOKYO

W.B. SAUNDERS COMPANY
A Division of Elsevier Inc.

Elsevier, Inc., 1600 John F. Kennedy Blvd., Suite 1800, Philadelphia, PA 19103-2899

http://www.vetexotic.theclinics.com

VETERINARY CLINICS OF NORTH AMERICA:	Volume 9, Number 1
EXOTIC ANIMAL PRACTICE	ISSN 1094-9194
JANUARY 2006	ISBN 1-4160-3466-8
Editor: John Vassallo	

Reprints. For copies of 100 or more of articles in this publication, please contact the commercial Reprints Department, Elsevier Inc., 360 Park Avenue South, New York, New York 10010-1710. Tel: (212) 633-3813 Fax: (212) 633-1935, e-mail: reprints@elsevier.com

The ideas and opinions expressed in *Veterinary Clinics of North America: Exotic Animal Practice* do not necessarily reflect those of the Publisher. The Publisher does not assume any responsibility for any injury and/or damage to persons or property arising out of or related to any use of the material contained in this periodical. The reader is advised to check the appropriate medical literature and the product information currently provided by the manufacturer of each drug to be administered to verify the dosage, the method and duration of administration, or contraindications. It is the responsibility of the treating physician or other health care professional, relying on independent experience and knowledge of the patient, to determine drug dosages and the best treatment for the patient. Mention of any product in this issue should not be construed as endorsement by the contributors, editors, or the Publisher of the product or manufacturers' claims.

Veterinary Clinics of North America: Exotic Animal Practice (ISSN 1094-9194) is published in January, May, and September by Elsevier, Inc.; Corporate and editorial offices: Elsevier, Inc., 1600 John F. Kennedy Blvd., Suite 1800, Philadelphia, PA 19103-2899. Accounting and circulation offices: 6277 Sea Harbor Drive, Orlando, FL 32887-4800. Subscription prices are $135.00 per year for US individuals, $230.00 per year for US institutions, $70.00 per year for US students and residents, $160.00 per year for Canadian individuals, $265.00 per year for Canadian institutions, $170.00 per year for international individuals, $265.00 per year for international institutions and $85.00 per year for Canadian and foreign students/residents. To receive student/resident rate, orders must be accompanied by name of affiliated institution, date of term, and the *signature* of program/residency coordinator on institution letterhead. Orders will be billed at individual rate until proof of status is received. Foreign air speed delivery is included in all *Clinics* subscription prices. All prices are subject to change without notice.

POSTMASTER: Send address changes to *Veterinary Clinics of North America: Exotic Animal Practice*; W.B. Saunders Company, Periodicals Fulfillment, Orlando, FL 32887-4800. **Customer Service: 1-800-654-2452 (US). From outside of the US, call 1-407-345-1000.**

Veterinary Clinics of North America: Exotic Animal Practice is covered in *Index Medicus*.

Printed in the United States of America.

CONSULTING EDITOR

AGNES E. RUPLEY, DVM, Diplomate, American Board of Veterinary Practitioners-Avian; and Director and Chief Veterinarian, All Pets Medical & Laser Surgical Center, College Station, Texas

GUEST EDITOR

M. SCOTT ECHOLS, DVM, American Board of Veterinary Practioners-Avian Practice; Westgate Pet and Bird Hospital, Austin, Texas

CONTRIBUTORS

TODD R. CECIL, DVM, Associate Veterinarian, Avian and Exotic Animal Hospital, San Diego, California

M. SCOTT ECHOLS, DVM, American Board of Veterinary Practioners-Avian Practice; Westgate Pet and Bird Hospital, Austin, Texas

PETER G. FISHER, DVM, Pet Care Veterinary Hospital, Virginia Beach, Virginia

STEPHEN J. HERNANDEZ-DIVERS, BVM, DZOOMED, MRCVS, RCVS, Specialist in Zoo and Wildlife Medicine; Diplomate, American College of Zoological Medicine; Associate Professor of Exotic Animal, Wildlife, and Zoological Medicine, Department of Small Animal Medicine and Surgery, College of Veterinary Medicine, University of Georgia, Athens, Georgia

PETER H. HOLZ, BVSc, DVSc, MACVSc, Diplomate, American College of Zoological Medicine; Healesville Sanctuary, Healesville, Victoria, Australia

CHRISTAL POLLOCK, DVM, American Board of Veterinary Practioners-Avian Practice; Associate, North Coast Bird and Exotic Specialties, Akron, Ohio; Formerly, Assistant Professor, College of Veterinary Medicine, Kansas State University, Manhattan, Kansas

SHANE R. RAIDAL, BVSc, PhD, FACVSc, Associate Professor in Veterinary Pathology, School of Veterinary and Biomedical Sciences, Murdoch University, Murdoch, Western Australia, Australia

SHARANNE L. RAIDAL, BVSc, MVSt, PhD, MACVSc, Senior Lecturer in Veterinary Pathology, School of Veterinary and Biomedical Sciences, Murdoch University, Murdoch, Western Australia, Australia

ROBERT E. SCHMIDT, DVM, PhD, Diplomate, American College of Veterinary Pathologists; Zoo/Exotic Pathology Service, Greenview, California

PAOLO SELLERI, Dr Med Vet, PhD, Centro Veterinario Specialistico—Animali Esotici, Rome, Italy; Dipartimento di Scienze Cliniche Veterinarie, Facoltà di Medicina Veterinaria, Legnaro, Padua, Italy

PEERNEL ZWART, DVM, PhD, Diplomate, European College of Veterinary Pathologists; Emeritus Professor, Department of Veterinary Pathology, State University, Utrecht, The Netherlands

CONTRIBUTORS

CONTENTS

include systemic antibiotics, diuretics, parenteral vitamin A, and agents to lower uric acid levels such as allopurinol.

GOAL STATEMENT

The goal of the *Veterinary Clinics of North America: Exotic Animal Practice* is to keep practicing veterinarians up to date with current clinical practice in exotic animal medicine by providing timely articles reviewing the state of the art in exotic animal care.

ACCREDITATION

The *Veterinary Clinics of North America: Exotic Animal Practice* offers continuing education credits, awarded by Cummings School of Veterinary Medicine at Tufts University, Office of Continuing Education.

Cummings School of Veterinary Medicine at Tufts University is a designated provider of continuing veterinary medical education. Veterinarians participating in this learning activity may earn up to 6 credits per issue up to a maximum of 18 credits per year. Credits awarded may not apply toward license renewal in all states. It is the responsibility of each participant to verify the requirements of their state licensing board.

Credit can be earned by reading the text material, taking the examination online at *http://www.theclinics.com/home/cme*, and completing the program evaluation. Following your completion of the test and program evaluation, and review of any and all incorrect answers, you may print your certificate.

TO ENROLL

To enroll in the *Veterinary Clinics of North America: Exotic Animal Practice* Continuing Veterinary Medical Education Program, call customer service at 1-800-654-2452 or sign up online at *http://www.theclinics.com/home/cme.* The CVME program is now available at a special introductory rate of $49.95 for a year's subscription.

FORTHCOMING ISSUES

RECENT ISSUES

VETERINARY
CLINICS
Exotic Animal Practice

Vet Clin Exot Anim 9 (2006) xi–xii

Preface

Renal Disease

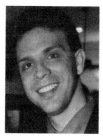

M. Scott Echols, DVM, DABVP-Avian Practice
Guest Editor

The veterinary and human medical literature frequently describes renal disease as a major cause of morbidity and mortality across the species. Of course, most of the emphasis has been focused on renal diseases in domestic animals (most notably cats and dogs) and in humans.

Ever since my residency began, I have had a strong interest in renal disease. When I graduated from veterinary school 10 years ago and began working in private practice, I found kidney diseases frustrating in exotic pets, mostly because there was little information on disease diagnosis, management, and treatment. Since that time, we have learned that many renal diseases in exotics can be diagnosed premortem, most can be managed when properly diagnosed before end stage, and some can be even "treated." Concurrently, the same can be said of domestic animal medicine.

I was honored when asked to put together this issue. More importantly, I am grateful to the outstanding authors who agreed to write articles. As you look through the table of contents, you probably will be familiar with the authors, many of whom are experienced lecturers and writers and are true experts in their respective fields. The cast of authors is as impressive as their works.

Please take the time to review these articles with the intention of understanding the types of renal disease and diagnostic methods available for the respective species. Once a proper diagnosis is made, management and treatment options are somewhat similar across species. Ultimately, the goal of this series is to improve the quality of life for the wonderful animals that are in our care.

doi:10.1016/j.cvex.2005.10.006

Again, my thanks to the authors for their time, effort, and most notably, expertise.

M. Scott Echols, DVM, DABVP-Avian Practice
Westgate Pet and Bird Hospital
4534 Westgate Boulevard, Suite 100, Austin, TX 78745, USA

E-mail address: spotdvm@aol.com

ELSEVIER
SAUNDERS

VETERINARY
CLINICS
Exotic Animal Practice

Vet Clin Exot Anim 9 (2006) 1–11

Comparative Renal Anatomy of Exotic Species

Peter H. Holz, BVSc, DVSc, MACVSc[a],
Shane R. Raidal, BVSc, PhD[b],*

[a]*Healesville Sanctuary, Healesville, Victoria 3777, Australia*
[b]*School of Veterinary and Biomedical Sciences, Murdoch University,
South Street, Murdoch, Western Australia 6150, Australia*

All living organisms consume nutrients that are required for the production of both tissue and energy. The waste products of this process include nitrogenous materials and inorganic salts. They are removed from the body by excretory organs, which in vertebrates have developed into kidneys and into salt glands in some birds and reptiles. Many invertebrates use a series of excretory organs called nephridia to perform the same function. As an example, the nephridia of the giant Gippsland earthworm (*Megascolides australis*) contain a ciliated funnel that opens into the coelomic cavity and connects to a tubule, which opens to the exterior of the body by a nephridiopore [1]. Coelomic fluid enters the tubule, water and important nutrients are absorbed through the wall, and dilute urine containing urea and ammonia is excreted from the tubule. Insects have a similar arrangement except that the tubules connect to the hindgut instead of the exterior. Body fluids are drawn from the coelom into these by osmosis following active secretion of sodium, potassium, and uric acid inside the tubule. Water is reabsorbed from the hindgut, and nitrogenous waste, mostly uric acid, is expelled in relatively dry feces.

Evolution of the kidney

Even though they perform similar functions, there is no evolutionary connection between invertebrate nephridia and vertebrate kidneys. Both evolved independently. The vertebrate kidney is derived from embryonic

---

* Corresponding author.
E-mail address: raidal@murdoch.edu.au (S.R. Raidal).

mesoderm. The progenitor of the current vertebrate kidney was the archinephros. The archinephros consisted of pairs of archinephric ducts located on the dorsal side of the body cavity that extended the length of the coelom. Each pair of ducts was joined by a series of segmentally arranged tubules, one pair of tubules to a segment. The tubules opened directly into the coelom via a ciliated funnel-shaped nephrostome (Fig. 1); associated with each nephrostome was a glomerulus. Blood entered the glomerulus by the afferent arteriole, which branched to form a series of interarterial capillaries. These combined to form the efferent arteriole, which drained blood from the glomerulus back into the general circulation. The knot of capillaries was surrounded by a double-walled structure called Bowman's capsule. Fluid passed from the glomerular capillaries into the coelom, in the case of external glomeruli, or into the cavity of Bowman's capsule, in the case of internal glomeruli. Cilia moved fluid from the coelom and Bowman's capsule into the tubule. Tubule cells also secreted wastes into the tubule lumen. Water and other constituents were absorbed farther along the tubule. This material then entered the archinephric duct and was excreted into the cloaca. The glomerulus, Bowman's capsule, and tubule are collectively known as the nephron.

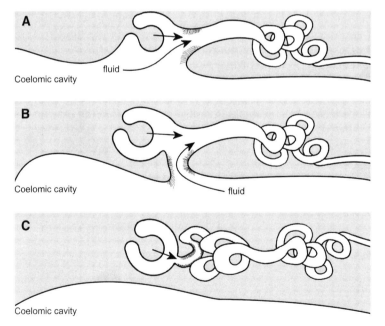

Fig. 1. Development of the nephron as glomeruli become internalized. (*A*) The nephridia of invertebrates and the pronephros of larval or embryonic vertebrates share a similar but evolutionarily distinct structure with a ciliated opening to the coelomic cavity (nephrostome) and an external glomerulus (glomus). (*B*) The mesonephros of many embryonic vertebrates and nephrons of adult caecilians possess a ciliated nephrostome and internalized glomerulus. (*C*) Typical internalized glomerulus of vertebrates, with many species retaining a ciliated epithelium.

A form of the ancestral archinephros still exists in some current species. It is divisible into two sections. The anterior part is the pronephros, which is the first-formed kidney of a vertebrate embryo and lies dorsal to the pericardial cavity. This pronephros is anatomically the same as the ancestral archinephros and still occurs functionally in hagfish (*Myxine* spp, *Neomyxine* spp, *Paramyxine* spp, and *Eptatretus* spp) and fish of the genera *Zoarces, Fierasfer,* and *Lepadogaster.* In fish it is also known as the "head kidney." The posterior section is called the opisthonephros and acts as the functional kidney in most fish and amphibians.

The opisthonephros, unlike the pronephros, does not contain segmentally arranged tubules. Numerous tubules may be contained within a single segment, and they have lost the direct connection with the coelom maintained by the pronephros. The tubules have differentiated into proximal and distal segments, which terminate in a collecting duct. The collecting ducts empty into the archinephric duct.

Reptiles, birds, and mammals possess three types of kidneys: the pronephros, mesonephros, and metanephros, which appear in succession in a cranio-caudal direction during embryonic development. Each of these embryonic kidneys lays the foundation for the induction of the next one. The pronephric primordium initially appears in the intermediate mesoderm located between the somites and the lateral plate mesoderm. The pronephros of birds has been considered nonfunctional, but more recent evidence indicates otherwise [2]. Nephrostomes are a characteristic feature of the mesonephric kidneys of freshwater vertebrates; they are still present in the stages of development of the mesonephric kidneys of birds and some mammals, such as the monotremes and elephant [3–5]. Kidney organogenesis progresses stepwise to the completion of metanephros development soon after birth, and only the metanephros persists to become the functional adult kidney [6]. Still, in reptiles and marsupials, the mesonephric kidney can provide significant functional capacity in the regulation of water and ion balance for at least a short time after birth [7].

The metanephros forms on either side of the body and is more compact than the preceding organs. The pronephros and mesonephros retain the archinephric duct, but this is termed the Wolffian duct while the mesonephros is functional. The duct degenerates when the metanephros forms and is replaced by the ureter, which begins as a diverticulum of the Wolffian duct. Tubule differentiation within the metanephros is similar to that in the opisthonephros but varies somewhat among the vertebrate groups. Basically, it consists of a neck segment, proximal tubule, intermediate segment, distal tubule, and collecting duct [8].

Fish

With some exceptions, the fish kidney is a single long, thin, fused organ lying retroperitoneally just ventral to the spinal column, occupying the dorsal wall of the coelomic cavity along its entire length. The kidney is to-pographically divided into the cranial kidney, which is the old pronephros, and the caudal kidney, which is the opisthonephros (Fig. 2). In some species, such as the channel catfish, goldfish, and marine angelfish, the cranial part of the kidney, which consists of endocrine and hematopoietic tissue, is phys-ically separate from the caudal part. In sharks and rays the kidneys have not fused but remain entirely separate [9].

The nephrons of a number of marine fish, such as sea horses, pipefish, and frogfish, lack glomeruli. Freshwater fish have larger and more numer-ous glomeruli than marine fish. The neck segment of the tubule is lined by a low cuboidal epithelium with long cilia. The proximal tubule may be divided into two segments: I and II. Segment I has an eosinophilic cuboidal to columnar epithelium with a distinct brush border and central or basal nuclei. Segment II has an acidophilic columnar epithelium with a central nucleus and prominent brush border. The intermediate segment is absent in many fish but well developed in carp. The epithelium is cuboidal and cil-iated, and the brush border becomes intermittent. Marine fish lack a distal tubule. In freshwater fish, the epithelial cells of the distal tubule are less eo-sinophilic than those of the proximal tubule and lack a brush border. The nephron is arranged perpendicular to the collecting duct, except in the lam-prey (*Lampetra fluviatilis*), where it is arranged parallel to it, as in mammals. The archinephric duct is lined with a columnar epithelial layer. In some fish, such as catfish, this duct may be enlarged distally to form a urinary bladder. This is a thin-walled sac lined by one or two layers of cuboidal to columnar epithelium.

Nephrons are only found in the caudal kidney (see Fig. 2). The cranial kidney contains lymphoid tissue, hematopoietic cells, and, in carp and gold-fish, thyroid follicles [10].

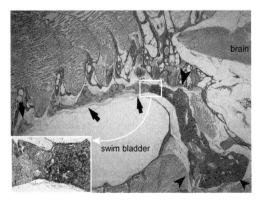

Fig. 2. A piscine kidney, outlining the anatomy of the predominantly lymphoid pronephros or "head kidney" (*arrowheads*) and its connection (*insert*) to the opisthonephros (*arrows*) or caudal kidney, which functions like other vertebrate kidneys.

Oxygenated blood flows from the gills into the dorsal aorta. The renal artery branches off the aorta and leads to the kidney. This vessel subdivides, becoming smaller and giving rise to the afferent arterioles that provide blood to the glomeruli. Blood leaves each glomerulus by the efferent arteriole and enters the capillary network that surrounds the tubule cells.

Venous blood enters the kidney by the caudal vein in the tail. The caudal vein divides into the right and left renal portal veins that pass along the dorsal aspect of the kidney, sending branches into the parenchyma. Segmental veins from the flank also empty into the renal portal veins. The renal portal veins provide blood to the renal tubules, which mixes with the blood coming from the efferent arterioles. This anatomic arrangement is present in a wide range of fish, including elasmobranchs, lungfish, sculpins, porcupinefish, balloonfish, mullets, sea robins, cusk-eels, goatfish, mackerels, polypterids, and soles [9]. Blood leaves the kidney by the caudal cardinal veins.

In cyprinids (eg, goldfish, koi, danios) and anguilliform eels, some blood passes through the renal portal system and some passes through the hepatic portal system [9]. This passage occurs through a connection between the caudal vein and the caudal intestinal vein. In eels, venous arcades pass between the renal portal veins and the intestinal vasculature.

In tench, cod, grenadiers, eelpouts, ide, daces, rudd, and some cyprinids, some blood goes from the caudal vein directly to the heart, bypassing the portal system [9]. In tench, only blood from the ventral portion of the tail goes through the kidneys. In the other fish, the caudal vein branches into a left renal portal vein that goes to the kidney and a right branch that goes directly to the heart.

In salmonids, perches, tunas, lumpfish, lumpsuckers, and freshwater fish, all the blood from the caudal vein goes directly to the heart, and the kidneys are supplied by segmental veins from the flank musculature. No blood goes through a portal system before travelling to the heart [9].

Amphibians

During amphibian metamorphosis, there may be a period during which the pronephros and the developing mesonephros function together. Prometamorphosis in green toads (*Bufo viridis*) results in paired kidneys, consisting of left and right cranial pronephroi that are found immediately behind the gills and cranial to two elongated mesonephroi. As in the invertebrate nephridia, the pronephroi contain tubules that open into the coelom via ciliated nephrostomes. Primary urine is formed on filtration from an external glomerulus and swept from the coelom into tubules [11].

The caecilian kidney is similar to that of fish in that it extends the length of the coelomic cavity. It is segmented. In caudates and anurans there are two separate kidneys found posteriorly and retroperitoneally. In hellbenders (*Cryptobranchus* sp), hynobid salamanders, and some anurans, such as tailed toads (*Ascaphus* sp), African ghost frogs (*Heleophryne* spp), and poison arrow frogs (*Dendrobates* spp), the kidneys are elongate, but in most species they are shorter, broader, and dorsoventrally flattened. A urinary bladder arises as a ventral diverticulum from the cloaca, a short distance beyond the openings of the archinephric ducts. In most amphibians the ducts enter the cloaca separately, but in some anurans, such as dwarf barking frogs (*Eleutherodactylus* spp), African ghost frogs (*Pachymedusa* sp), African striped frogs (*Kassina* spp), and many species of toad (*Bufo* spp), the ducts unite and enter through a single aperture. The ducts do not communicate directly with the bladder. Consequently, urine passes into the cloaca and is then forced into the bladder. Urine is expelled intermittently by opening the cloaca and contracting the muscular wall of the bladder. Some water is resorbed through the bladder wall.

The dorsal aorta leaves the heart, and several short renal arteries branch off into the dorsal aspect of the kidneys. The surface of the ventral kidney is supplied by the superficial renal artery, which emerges from the posterior oviductal artery just posterior to the kidney.

The veins of the hindlimb combine (along with the caudal vein in salamanders) to form the paired Jacobson's or renal portal veins that pass anteriorly on the dorsolateral surface of the kidney, from which they receive many small vessels. The renal portal veins then enter the postcaval vein [12].

Reptiles

In most lizards the kidneys are located deep in the pelvic canal. Monitors are the exception; their kidneys rest in the caudal coelom. The kidneys are paired, symmetric, elongated, slightly lobulated, and flattened dorsoventrally. In many species the caudal aspect of the kidneys is fused. They are completely separate in chameleons. A fully developed urinary bladder is present in slow worms, iguanas, geckos, chameleons, and the common blue-tongued skink (*Tiliqua scincoides*). A rudimentary bladder exists in ameivas, tegus, and whiptails. The kidneys of the tuatara (*Sphenodon punctatus*) are similar to those of lizards. They are paired, single lobed, crescent shaped, and tucked high in the dorsal wall of the pelvic canal. The two kidneys meet posteriorly but do not fuse. A bladder is present. Snake kidneys are paired, flattened, and elongated organs containing 25 to 30 lobules, except for in the dwarf boas (*Trophidophis* spp) and the rough boas (*Trachyboas* spp), whose kidneys are not lobulated. The right kidney lies cranial to the left. Snakes have no urinary bladder.

Chelonian kidneys are paired and lie in the caudal coelom just ventral to the carapace. Methods describing the ultrasonographic and endoscopic examination of chelonid kidneys have been described [13,14]. In marine turtles, the kidneys are cranial to the pelvic girdle, symmetric and flattened, lobulated, and closely applied to the posterior wall of the pleuroperitoneal cavity. In the green sea turtle (*Chelonia mydas*), the ability to differentiate new functional nephrons is retained for at least 5 years after hatching [15]. The functional nephron includes a glomerulus, proximal tubule, intermediate segment, distal convoluted tubule, and collecting tubule [15]. Ureters leave the kidneys and enter the urinary bladder, as in mammals. The bladder is connected to the cloaca via the urethra. Crocodilians have paired lobulated kidneys that lie against the dorsal body wall adjacent to the spinal column. The left kidney may be larger than the right. Crocodilians have no urinary bladder [16,17].

Structurally, reptilian glomeruli are poorly developed, with a lower number of capillaries per gram body weight than those of birds. All the tubule segments except the distal tubule consist of ciliated, cuboidal cells. The cells of the distal tubule lack cilia.

The distal tubule is followed by the sex segment. In all female reptiles and male chelonians, this consists of columnar mucus-secreting cells. In male snakes and lizards, the cells are flat and filled with mucous during the nonbreeding season. During the breeding season these cells increase two to four times in height and are filled with large refractile granules that stain brightly eosinophilic with hematoxylin and eosin. They contain acid phosphatase, phospholipids, glycoprotein, mucoprotein, and amino acids. The function of the secretions contained within the sex segment is unknown. A number of theories have been proposed: for instance, the secretions may act to produce a copulatory plug to prevent rivals from mating successfully. Alternatively, they may block the tubules during copulation to keep the semen and the urine separate, or they may be a source of energy for the sperm.

After the sex segment, the nephron finishes with the collecting duct. These cells are similar to those contained in the sex segment, except that mucus is only present at the tip of the cell. The collecting ducts are oriented at right angles to the long axis of the kidney. They originate on the dorsolateral surface of each lobule, wrap around the lateral margin of the lobule, and pass ventrally into the ureter, which lies on the ventromedial surface of the kidney.

Arterial blood is supplied by a variable number of renal arteries branching off the aorta. Venous anatomy is similar among the four reptile groups. In lizards, blood flows from the tail by the caudal vein and from the hind legs by the iliac veins and then enters two afferent renal portal veins that convey it to the kidneys. However, angiography studies in green iguanas (*Iguana iguana*) have shown that most blood returning from the pelvic limb can bypass the kidney and enter the general circulation [18]. In the kidneys, the blood enters a series of capillaries that perfuse the renal tubule cells. From there the blood leaves the kidneys by the efferent renal portal veins. These fuse to form the postcaval vein, which conveys the blood back to the heart. Pelvic veins connect to the iliac veins before their attachment with the afferent renal portal veins and may divert blood around the kidneys into the single abdominal vein. From here the blood flows to the liver.

Venous blood flow in snakes is similar except for the absence of iliac veins. Blood is able to bypass the kidneys through the mesenteric vein, which receives connections directly from the afferent renal portal veins. The mesenteric venous blood is carried to the liver. The abdominal vein is present but is only connected to the afferent renal portal veins in the African rock python (*Python sebae*). In other species it has its origin in the fat bodies.

The tuatara is similar to lizards, but there is no direct connection between the iliac veins and the abdominal vein. It has been hypothesized that a connection to the abdominal vein may exist within the body of the kidneys. Chelonians and crocodilians have two abdominal veins, which are linked by a transverse anastomosis in the former group. In crocodilians, the abdominal veins are connected to the iliac vein, and, as in snakes, a mesenteric vein originates from the afferent renal portal veins.

Birds

The avian kidney is larger than the kidneys of mammals of similar body size, composing 1% to 2.6% of avian body weight compared with only 0.5% of mammalian body weight. Bird kidneys lie symmetrically in the renal fossae, which are bony depressions in the synsacrum. They extend as far as the lungs cranially and to the end of the synsacrum caudally. They are covered by a thin peritoneal serosa; in fat birds there may be abundant adipose tissue around the kidneys, but they are usually surrounded by an invagination of the abdominal airsac.

Each kidney is divided into cranial, middle, and caudal divisions or lobes that are supplied by major blood vessels. There are 13 to 17 lobules, separated by interlobular veins, in each lobe, and "cortical" tissue predominates. Each "medulla" receives collecting ducts from several adjacent lobules. In most passerines, the middle and caudal lobes are fused. Only the caudal lobes are fused in herons, puffins, and penguins. Hornbills lack a middle lobe.

The collecting ducts coalesce to form medullary collecting ducts. These ducts then combine from several adjacent lobules into a single cone-shaped collecting duct. The lobules that drain into this duct together form a renal lobe. These large collecting ducts coalesce to form the ureter. The ureter is thus branched to service each medullary cone. The ureter lies on the surface of the kidney in association with the blood vessels, except in the cranial division where it is embedded in the kidney, and distally it empties into the cloaca. There is no urinary bladder [19]. However, in ostriches the coprodeum functions like a urinary bladder, and final modification of urinary solutes can occur here [20].

Birds have two types of nephrons. The cortical nephron is similar to the reptilian nephron because it lacks a loop of Henle, has a short intermediate segment, and is oriented perpendicular to the collecting duct. The medullary nephron has a loop of Henle inserted between the proximal and distal tubules and is similar to mammalian nephrons, being arranged parallel to the collecting ducts. In the different species, proportions of mammalian-type nephrons vary from 10% in Gambel's quail (*Callipepla gambelii*) up to 30% in European starlings (*Sturnus vulgaris*). The appearance of a loop of Henle means that birds, like mammals, can produce urine that is hypertonic compared with blood [21].

The kidney is provided with arterial blood by the cranial, middle, and caudal renal arteries, which provide blood to the cranial, middle, and caudal kidney lobes, respectively. These branch to form intralobular arteries, which give rise to the afferent arterioles. The efferent arterioles empty into the peritubular capillary plexus, which drains into the intralobular veins.

The cranial and caudal renal portal veins form a ring that encompasses both kidneys by joining the external iliac and caudal renal veins. Venous blood enters this ring by the internal vertebral venous sinus, the caudal mesenteric vein, the external iliac veins, the ischiadic veins, and the internal iliac veins. The afferent renal branches leave this ring and penetrate the renal parenchyma where they become the interlobular veins, which drain into the peritubular capillary plexus. From here blood enters the intralobular veins, efferent renal veins, and finally the cranial and caudal renal veins. These open into the common iliac vein [17].

The renal portal valve is situated within the common iliac vein. When this valve is open, blood is diverted away from the kidneys into the caudal vena cava, and when it is closed, blood is shunted through the kidneys (Fig. 3). The valve is inhibited by adrenaline and stimulated by acetylcholine [19].

Mammals

The mammalian kidney is bean shaped, attached to the dorsal body wall, and retroperitoneal. It is divided into cortex and medulla. The cortex contains the nephrons; the collecting ducts are found in the medulla. This basic design constitutes the unipapillate kidney found in mammals weighing less than 5 kg. Larger mammals have developed a medulla of decreased depth but increased length. This is the crest kidney found in carnivores and some artiodactylids, such as camels and wildebeests. In primates, the medulla is divided into a series of lobes, whereas the cortex remains undivided, forming the compound multireniculate kidney. The largest mammals have a divided cortex as well as a divided medulla. This discrete multireniculate kidney is found in proboscids (elephants), pinnipeds (seals and walruses), cetaceans (whales and porpoises), and some artiodactylids (eg, cattle, deer, camels). A urinary bladder is present in all species. In all but the monotremes (platypus and echidna), the ureters enter the bladder dorsally. The bladder is connected externally by means of the urethra. In monotremes, the ureters connect directly to the urogenital sinus, opposite the neck of

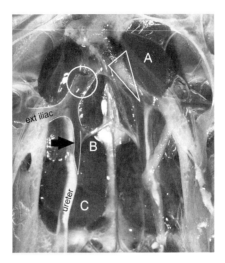

Fig. 3. The avian kidney, demonstrating the cranial (*A*), middle (*B*), and caudal (*C*) lobes. The outlines of the external iliac vein (ext iliac), the caudal renal vein (*arrow*), and the common iliac vein are shown. The position of the renal portal valve within the common iliac vein is circled. When this valve is open, blood is diverted away from the kidneys into the caudal vena cava, and when it is closed blood is shunted through the kidneys. The position of the ovary is outlined (*triangle*).

the bladder. The sinus connects to the cloaca. In most mammals the cloaca is divided into two parts, each having an independent opening to the outside. The dorsal portion is the rectum and the ventral portion is the urogenital sinus. This division does not occur in monotremes or marsupials [22].

The mammalian nephron follows the basic pattern. However, there is no neck segment. The proximal tubule is lined by an acidophilic cuboidal epithelium with a brush border and central nuclei. This is followed by the loop of Henle, which consists of a thin descending segment followed by a thick ascending segment. The thin segment is lined with a squamous epithelium. The thick segment and distal tubule are both lined with a cuboidal epithelium, but the cells are less acidophilic than those in the proximal tubule and lack the brush border. The collecting duct is lined by cuboidal epithelial cells, which gradually become columnar as they penetrate into the medulla [23].

Arterial blood reaches the kidneys by the renal arteries, which branch off the aorta. Accessory renal arteries may come from the caudal mesenteric, testicular, ovarian, and deep circumflex iliac arteries that enter the caudal part of the kidney. The renal arteries form arcuate arteries, which send branches into the cortex and medulla. The cortical vessels have a radial course and give off branches that become the afferent arterioles. The medullary branches descend into the renal pyramids. The afferent arterioles form the glomeruli and then the efferent arterioles, which lead into the capillaries that surround the tubules. These then lead into the renal veins, which empty into the caudal vena cava. There is no renal portal circulation [24].

References

[1] Spencer WB. The anatomy of *Megascolides australis*. Transactions of the Royal Society of Victoria 1888;1(1):3–60.

[2] Keibel F. In: Semon R, editor. Zoologische Forschungreisen in Australien und dem Malayischen Archipel. Jena (Germany): Fischer; 1904. p. 3:51–3:206.

[3] van der Schoot P. Foetal genital development in *Hyrax capensis*, a species with primary testicondia: proposal for the evolution of Hunter's gubernaculum. Anat Rec 1996;244: 386–401.

[4] Gaeth AP, Short RV, Renfree MB. The developing renal, reproductive, and respiratory systems of the African elephant suggest an aquatic ancestry. Proc Natl Acad Sci USA 1999;96: 5555–8.

[5] Bouchard M. Transcriptional control of kidney development. Differentiation 2004;72: 295–306.

[6] Beuchat CA, Braun EJ. Allometry of the kidney: implications for the ontogeny of osmoregulation. Am J Physiol 1988;255:760–7.

[7] Hiruma T, Nakamura H. Origin and development of the pronephros in the chick embryo. J Anat 2003;203(6):539–52.

[8] Weichert CK. Excretory system. In: Anatomy of the chordates. 4th edition. New York: McGraw-Hill; 1970. p. 250–73.

[9] Stoskopf MK. Anatomy. In: Fish medicine. Philadelphia: WB Saunders; 1993. p. 2–30.

[10] Stoskopf MK. Fish histology. In: Fish medicine. Philadelphia: WB Saunders; 1993. p. 31–47.

[11] Mobjerg N, Larsen EH, Jespersen A. Morphology of the kidney in larvae of *Bufo viridis* (Amphibia, Anura, Bufonidae). J Morphol 2000;245(3):177–95.

[12] Duellman WE, Trueb L. Integumentary, sensory, and visceral systems. In: Biology of amphibians. Baltimore (MD): Johns Hopkins University Press; 1986. p. 367–414.

[13] Martorell J, Espada Y, Ruiz de Gopegui R. Normal echoanatomy of the red-eared slider terrapin (*Trachemys scripta elegans*). Vet Rec 2004;155(14):417–20.

[14] Hernandez-Divers SJ. Endoscopic renal evaluation and biopsy of Chelonia. Vet Rec 2004; 154(3):73–80.

[15] Solomon SE. The morphology of the kidney of the green turtle (*Chelonia mydas*). J Anat 1985;140:355–69.

[16] Fox H. The urogenital system of reptiles. In: Gans C, editor. Biology of the reptilia, Vol. 6. New York: Academic Press; 1977. p. 1–157.

[17] Canny C. Gross anatomy and imaging of the avian and reptilian urinary system. Semin Avian Exotic Pet Med 1998;7:72–80.

[18] Benson KG, Forrest L. Characterization of the renal portal system of the common green iguana (*Iguana iguana*) by digital subtraction imaging. J Zoo Wildl Med 1999;30(2):235–41.

[19] King AS, McLelland J. Urinary system. In: Birds, their structure and function. 2nd edition. Eastbourne (UK): Bailliere Tindall; 1984. p. 175–86.

[20] Deeming DC. Physiology. In: The ostrich: biology, production and health. Wallingford and Oxon (UK): CABI Publishing; 1999. p. 54–60.

[21] Dantzler WH. Comparative aspects of renal function. In: Seldin DW, Giebisch G, editors. The kidney: physiology and pathophysiology. New York: Raven Press; 1985. p. 333–64.

[22] Braun EJ. Comparative renal function in reptiles, birds and mammals. Semin Avian Exotic Pet Med 1998;7:62–71.

[23] Junqueira LC, Carneiro J. Urinary system. In: Basic histology. 3rd edition. Los Altos (CA): Lange Medical Publications; 1980. p. 392–409.

[24] Getty R. The anatomy of the domestic animals. 5th edition. Philadelphia: WB Saunders; 1975.

VETERINARY
CLINICS
Exotic Animal Practice

ELSEVIER
SAUNDERS

Vet Clin Exot Anim 9 (2006) 13–31

Comparative Renal Physiology of Exotic Species

Shane R. Raidal, BVSc, PhD*,
Sharanne L. Raidal, BVSc, MVSt, PhD, MACVSc

School of Veterinary and Biomedical Sciences, Murdoch University, South Street, Murdoch, Western Australia, 6150 Australia

In this article the osmoregulatory, acid-base homeostasis, and excretory functions of the renal system of invertebrates and vertebrates are reviewed and summarized. The mammalian renal system is the most highly evolved in terms of the range of functions performed by the kidneys, including the urine concentration capacity that may be achieved without further (post-renal) modification of urine. As such, mammalian renal physiology is appropriately the main model learned by veterinarians. However, renal physiology in other animals can be very different, and a sound knowledge of these differences is important for understanding health and disease processes that involve the kidneys, as well as ion and water homeostasis. Many animals rely on multiple organs, such as gills and skin, along with the kidneys to maintain osmotic, ionic, and pH balance and nitrogenous waste excretion. The relative importance of the renal system therefore varies depending on the species and its natural habitat. Some animals rely heavily on postrenal modification of urine to conserve water and salt balance; this reliance can confer biologic advantages under certain environmental conditions, as well as influence the interpretation of disease signs and treatment modalities.

Body fluid regulation and nitrogenous waste excretion

Given the range of animals that the exotic veterinarian may encounter, any discussion of renal nitrogenous waste excretion, osmoregulation, acid-base balance, and other physiologic roles of the renal system should recognize that many animals employ multiorgan mechanisms to maintain osmotic,

* Corresponding author.
E-mail address: raidal@murdoch.edu.au (S.R. Raidal).

1094-9194/06/$ - see front matter © 2006 Elsevier Inc. All rights reserved.
doi:10.1016/j.cvex.2005.09.002
vetexotic.theclinics.com

ionic, and pH homeostasis and nitrogenous waste excretion. Marine reptiles and birds possess nasal glands that excrete salt (sodium [Na$^+$] and chlorine [Cl$^-$] ions), and sharks have rectal glands that perform a similar function. Gills and the opercular epithelium are important excretory and osmoregulatory organs in aquatic invertebrates and fish [1], whereas in birds, reptiles, and amphibians there is considerable postrenal modification of urine (Fig. 1). In contrast, there is no postrenal modification of mammalian urine, and other solute secretory organs are redundant. This condition is possible because of the enhanced urine osmotic concentrating capacity achieved by the differentiation of renal cortex and medulla and the development of the loop of Henle (Table 1). The mammalian kidney is thus an efficient primary

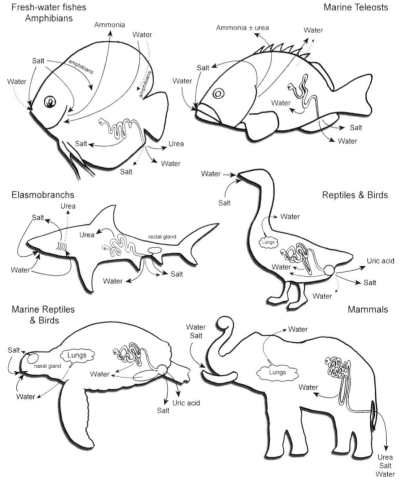

Fig. 1. Major electrolytes, water movement, and the role of renal and extrarenal mechanisms in the different classes of vertebrates.

Table 1
Plasma ionic concentrations and renal concentrating ability in various species

	Na (mM)	Cl (mM)	K (mM)	Mg (mM)	Ca (mM)	SO₄ (mM)	Urea (mM)	TMAO (mM)	Total osmolality (mOsm)	Glomeruler filtration rate	Urine osmolality (mOsm)	USG
Seawater	439	513	9.3	50	9.6	26	—	—	1050			
Hagfish [78]	537	542	9.1	18	5.9	6.3			1035			
Shark [78]	286	246	6.0	3.0	5.0	0.5	441	71	1018	3.5 mL/kg/h	780 [78]	
Marine fish	180	196	5.1	2.5	2.8	2.7		—	452	0.5 mL/kg/h	≅450	
Freshwater	0.25	0.25	0.005	0.04	0.07	0.05			1			
Freshwater fish	130	125	2.9	1.2	2.1	—	—	—	274	4 mL/kg/h	20	
Amphibian [79]	108	76	2.4	0.6	2	2	—	—	234		≤230	
Reptile[a] [80]	145	110	4.5	1.3	2.5		<100 mg/L	—	310	1.5–5 mL/kg/h[b]		
Bird[a] [80,81]	150	114	4.5	0.9	2.5		—	—	320	52–170 mL/kg/h[b,c]		
Human [68]	142	108	4.2	0.8	1.3	0.5	4	—	302	120 mL/min [6]	1200 [6]	<1.020
Dog	145	114	4.5	0.84	2.5		6.1	—	295		2000	<1.030
Dolphin	155	120	3.6	0.65	2.3		16.7	—	340 [68]		1815 [68]	<1.075
Desert opossum[d]											9015[d]	

Unless otherwise indicated values are taken from Evans [77].

Abbreviations: TMAO, trimethylamine N-oxide; USG, urine specific gravity.

[a] Values given are midpoint of reference range and will vary between species [80].

[b] Glomerular filtration rate (GFR) typical of control values reported [54] for a range of species: including dester and freshwater *Testudines, Crocodylus johnsoni,* and xeric lizards; snakes, lizards from mesic habitats had GFR closer to 15 mL/kg/h; saltwater crocodiles (*Crocodylus porosus*) had the lowest reported control GFR of 1.5 mL/kg/h.

[c] Control value for *Gallus domesticus* [54].

[d] Diaz et al [71] value cited is maximum urinary concentration reported for a marsupial and consistent with values obtained from similarly sized desert rodents.

organ of osmoregulation and excretion, which has evolved to perform four primary functions: the removal of nitrogenous wastes, the regulation of water balance and blood pressure, electrolyte homeostasis (particularly Na^+, potassium $[K^+]$, Cl^-, and calcium $[Ca^+]$ ions), and acid-base homeostasis. These four key functions are interrelated and serve to regulate plasma ion concentrations within the narrow limits required to maintain extracellular fluid (ECF) and intracellular fluid (ICF) volume and ionic composition. The mammalian kidney also has important endocrine roles, such as the secretion of erythropoietin, calcitrol, and renin.

Elimination of nitrogenous wastes

Ammonia (NH_3) is a byproduct of amino acid metabolism; because it is a base, it rapidly accepts an H^+ ion to form ammonium (NH_4^+) at physiologic pH [2]. Both NH_3 and NH_4^+ are toxic, and an effective excretion system is essential to maintaining cellular function. Hydrated NH_4^+ has the same ionic radius as the hydrated K^+ ion. Because of its K^+–like behavior, NH_4^+ can affect the membrane potential of neurons and other cells [3,4] and result in toxic accumulations of glutamine and disruption of essential cellular functions. Across the animal kingdom, the ammonia concentration of body fluids is typically low (50–400 μmol/L) [4–6], and concentrations exceeding 1 mmol/L total ammonia (NH_3 and NH_4^+) are usually toxic to mammalian cells [7]. Animals may be classed as ammonotelic, ureotelic, or uricotelic, depending on whether they predominantly excrete ammonia or the more metabolically expensive but less toxic urea or uric acid, respectively. However, this distinction may be loose, because many have the capacity to excrete nitrogenous wastes in more than one form, or even in all three when conditions are appropriate.

Invertebrates

The renal function of invertebrates is primarily related to nitrogenous waste excretion. Most marine invertebrates are osmoconformers and may thus avoid the energy-expensive osmoregulation mechanisms required by vertebrates. Ammonia is the main nitrogenous waste excreted by aquatic invertebrates; its excretion via the gills in marine crustaceans is achieved by passive diffusion and active Na^+:NH_4^+ exchange [8]. In contrast, terrestrial arthropods, except for land crabs, primarily excrete purines, such as uric acid, xanthine, and guanine, and many can accumulate excretory material such as uric acid in internal organs and tissues until conditions are favorable for excretion [9–11]. Most crabs are ammonotelic regardless of their habitat; thus terrestrial crabs are forced to use various mechanisms to store and excrete ammonia effectively when their hydration status permits excretion [6].

Renal function in vertebrates

Osmoregulation and water balance in vertebrates are achieved by variation in water flux into or out of the body and the regulation of plasma ionic composition, particularly Na^+—although K^+ regulation is coupled to Na^+ at a number of levels and hence must also be considered. In terrestrial vertebrates, the need for increased water intake is perceived as thirst, mediated by the hypothalamus in response to neural input from oropharyngeal receptors (dry mucosa), increased plasma oncotic pressure, and increased angiotensin II concentrations secondary to decreased blood pressure. Water uptake across the integument is an important aspect of fluid homeostasis for amphibians. Fluid losses occur through the gastrointestinal and urinary tracts, along with insensible losses through the respiratory and integumentary systems.

Evidence of renin angiotensin systems (RAS) that contribute to osmoregulation, ionoregulation, and the control of blood circulation may be found in most vertebrates [12,13], and elements of the system can also be found in invertebrates [14]. Granulated juxtaglomerular cells similar to the renin-containing cells of the mammalian nephron are found in most extant vertebrate species, although not in agnathans (jawless fish) [12,13]. Prolonged hypovolemic hypotension or sodium depletion increases renin levels. Angiotensins elicit drinking, promote antidiuretic hormone (arginine vasopressin [AVP] or arginine vasotocin [AVT]) release, and stimulate transepithelial ion transport. Secretion of the adrenal mineralocorticoid aldosterone is directly stimulated by angiotensin II, adrenocorticotropic hormone, and elevated K^+ in blood (mammals). Direct steroidogenic and antidiuretic hormone-releasing effects that promote mineral and fluid conservation are best developed in mammals (see later discussion).

Fish

Marine fish can only excrete urine that is isosmotic with plasma, and piscine kidneys tend to be small compared with those of other vertebrates. This difference reflects the greater importance that other organs, most notably the gills, have in nitrogenous waste excretion, ionic regulation, and water balance in an aquatic environment. In some species, such as the lungfish (*Arapaima gigas*), which transforms as an adult to become an almost obligate air-breather, the kidneys become greatly enlarged to cope with the added demands that result following branchial atrophy [15]. The kidneys of freshwater fish are larger than those of marine fish because, to maintain osmotic balance, freshwater fish must excrete a relatively large volume of dilute urine [16] with almost complete resorption of Na^+ and Cl^- from the proximal and distal tubules without the osmotic accompaniment of water (see Table 1).

Many extant fish are aglomerular; they achieve urine flow within the proximal tubule by the transepithelial active secretion of Cl^- and thus by passive diffusion of Na^+ and water into the lumen [17]. The importance of this mechanism in the filtering kidney is sometimes overlooked; the recurrent loss of piscine glomeruli throughout evolution suggests a mechanism of aglomerular urine formation intrinsic to renal tubules [17]. The distal nephron has low water permeability, and urine flow is determined largely by blood pressure, glomerular filtration rate, and circulating catecholamines.

Most fish are ammonotelic, and the gills are the primary site of ammonia excretion. Some are facultatively ureotelic when energy balance or other conditions are favorable [18], but even then most urea excretion is through the gills [19]. For example, urea synthesis and the percentage of total nitrogen excreted as urea may increase by as much as 60% in the slender African lungfish (*Protopterus dolloi*) after feeding [20], and this dampens the postprandial plasma ammonia surge that is well recognized in ammonotelic teleosts (higher bony fish).

Marine elasmobranchs (sharks, skates, rays, and sawfish) actively maintain high serum urea concentrations [21–23] in the 300 to 600 mM range [24,25] and thus risk the detrimental effects that urea can have on protein function [26]. Specialized adaptations to the gill epithelial cell membranes and active urea transport promote reabsorption of urea against a huge blood-to-water diffusion gradient [24]. Sharks withstand such high internal urea concentrations by accumulating methylamines and other low-molecular-weight osmolytes that offset the effects of urea on proteins [23,27]. Methylamines also have a protective role in the medulla of the mammalian kidney, where urea concentrations are high, but, like urea, they provide sharks with the added benefit of having considerably lower density than other body solutes. Most elasmobranchs, even euryhaline species such as the bull shark (*Carcharhinus leucas*), have plasma that is approximately isosmotic to seawater (see Table 1), approximately three times more concentrated than the plasma of all other vertebrates, and they lack a swim bladder. The positive buoyancy effect of high concentrations of plasma urea and methylamine helps them to maintain neutral buoyancy. Sharks also have a rectal gland that is important for maintaining salt balance, because the secretion is salt rich (500 mM) and urea poor (18 mM) but is isotonic with plasma [28].

Endocrine and neuroendocrine regulation of renal function in fish is not dissimilar to that reported for other vertebrates, but it is closely linked to the function of other sites of osmoregulation, particularly the branchial arch and gill epithelium. Fish, like all vertebrates, have a neurohypophysis, which is continuous with the floor of the diencephalon, and an adenohypophysis, which is derived from nonneural tissue [29]. Neurohypophyseal hormones are released into general circulation or into a portal system, depending on the species. Of the 10 neurohypophyseal hormones reported in other species, seven (AVT, glumitocin, aspartocin, valitocin, isotocin, oxytocin, and mesotocin) have been reported in fish [29]. The precise function of these peptides has not been fully elucidated, but most have effects on blood pressure and fluid control. For example, AVT and isotocin have a diuretic or antidiuretic effect, depending on experimental method. Like AVP in mammals, AVT probably has an antidiuretic effect in physiologic concentrations, primarily through a reduction in glomerular perfusion and glomerular filtration rate (GFR) [30,31]. But receptors are widely distributed through many organs, and AVT's precise functions and mechanism of action have not been determined [32,33].

Other neuroendocrine tissues are present in jawed fishes (chondrichthyans and osteichthyans). These have a neurohemal organ composed of large neurons (Dahlgren cells) in the caudal part of the spinal cord and, in most teleosts, the urophysis, a well-developed neurosecretory system extending ventrally from the spinal cord. The major products of these caudal neurosecretory systems are urotensins. Urotensin I (UI) is structurally homologous to corticotrophin-releasing hormone, and urotensin II (UII) demonstrates structural homology with somatostatins. Both have myotropic actions and osmoregulatory effects, UI probably by stimulation of steroid synthesis in the interrenal cells [29] and UII by regulating ion exchange across nonrenal epithelia [34].

Fish lack discrete adrenal glands; instead, steroids and catecholamines are synthesized by interrenal tissue, located in the pronephros or on the surface of the kidneys [29]. Cortisol is the major steroid produced, although there are traces of other corticosteroids and the mineralocorticoid aldosterone. In fish, by contrast with terrestrial vertebrates, the role of corticosteroids in ionic regulation is substantial and is primarily mediated through effects on the chloride cells of the branchial arch and the rectal gland in chondrichthyans.

Angiotensin II is the major product of the renin-angiotensin-aldosterone system in fish and sharks [35,36], as well as in higher vertebrates. As for mammals, enzymic activation of different products of this system occurs by means of renin, released from renal juxtaglomerular cells, and angiotensin-converting enzyme, which is more widely distributed in fish than in other species. In all major groups of fish, with the exception of agnathans, angiotensin II has roles in body fluid control and interrenal steroidogenesis analogous to those reported in higher vertebrates:

- Increased systemic blood pressure (an indirect effect mediated by catecholamines)
- Increased corticoid and mineralocorticoid secretion
- Increased drinking (especially in seawater teleosts)
- Reduced GFR (shown to be important in the adaptation of euryhaline teleosts to increased salinity) [37]

The teleost kidney is both an erythropoietic and erythropoietin-producing organ [38,39], but other organs, including the heart, liver, and brain, may be more important erythropoietin-secreting organs in some fish species [40]. Other endocrine functions of the piscine kidney include synthesis of stanniocalcin and insulin-like growth factors [29]. Stanniocalcin is produced by corpuscles of Stannius, which are usually paired and located within or on the kidneys. This hormone is a glycoprotein unique to osteichthyans and without clear homology to other hormones. It functions to prevent hypercalcemia in an aquatic environment, probably by acting as a calcium channel blocker at the gills. Evidence exists of a vitamin D_3 system in fish, but its role in calcium homeostasis, especially in renal regulation of calcium ion excretion, is unclear.

Finally, as observed in mammalian kidneys, fishes' renal function may be modulated by natriuretic peptides. These compounds have been demonstrated in agnathans, chondrichthyans, and teleosts. As in higher vertebrates, synthesis and release are controlled by factors related to increased blood volume, such as atrial or ventricular distension and increased plasma Na^+ concentrations or osmolality. Other hormones, such as glucocorticoids, thyroid hormone, angiotensin II, and endothelins, may also influence natriuretic peptide concentrations. Not surprisingly in an aquatic environment, the action of natriuretic peptides seems more related to salt regulation than to control of fluid volume and is more important in marine than in freshwater fish. Consistent with the lesser renal contribution to osmoregulation in fish, the effects of these peptides are probably mediated more directly through regulation of NaCl excretion by the rectal gland of elasmobranchs or Cl^- secretion across the gills in other fish.

Amphibians

Amphibians have three principal osmoregulatory organs: the kidneys, the urinary bladder, and the skin, which contribute to the regulation of plasma and body fluid composition [41,42]. Amphibians inhabit a range of aqueous and terrestrial environments; although the kidneys of all anurans are similar at the gross morphologic level, their nephron structure appears to be related to habitat [43]. The nephrons of aquatic species have a long and well-developed proximal segment and a relatively short distal segment. In contrast, terrestrial species have a long and well-developed distal segment. The peptide hormone angiotensin II stimulates cutaneous drinking in a similar manner to oral drinking in other vertebrate classes. Transcutaneous evaporative water loss is high in amphibians. Unsurprisingly, terrestrial amphibians are more tolerant of dehydration than other vertebrates, with some terrestrial species able to tolerate as much as 50% of total body water loss. Systemic tolerance of hyperosmolarity is seen, and plasma volume is preferentially conserved over ECF and ICF loss. The urinary bladder is an important site of water storage in these animals. The Australian water-holding frog (*Cyclorana platycephala*) can store large volumes of dilute urine in the urinary bladder, which offset evaporative losses during arid periods [44]. Bladder epithelial water permeability is regulated by AVT. Toads appear to be able to detect the presence of water in their bladders in addition to the availability of water in their environment, and dehydrated toads rapidly rehydrate by coordinating behavioral and physiologic mechanisms to enhance cutaneous water absorption [45].

Reptiles

The kidneys of reptiles are the chief site of osmoregulation and nitrogenous waste excretion, excepting those of marine reptiles, which possess salt glands. However, there is postrenal modification of urine in the cloaca or the urinary bladder or both (in those reptiles that have one). AVT is present in reptiles; AVT receptors are present in both the short intermediate segment of the nephron and the branched collecting duct system in the agamid lizard *Ctenophorus ornatus* [46]. Reptilian nephrons have an incipient juxtaglomerular apparatus, aglomerular nephrons, and a thin, short intermediate segment that connects the proximal and distal convoluted tubules. AVT may have a dual effect in the reptilian kidney, first diluting the urinary fluid in the thin intermediate segment, before it enters the collecting duct system, and then facilitating water reabsorption along an osmotic gradient as the urine passes through the final segments of the nephron. The intermediate segment may thus prove to be the evolutionary homologue of the thin-ascending limb of the loop of Henle in the mammalian kidney.

The distal tubules are longer in reptiles adapted to dry environments, and tubular reabsorption of fluid is primarily from the distal segments of the nephron. In freshwater turtles, the diuretic furosemide produces diuresis by doubling urine volume and increasing Na^+, Cl^-, and K^+ excretion principally by inhibiting tubular reabsorption in the distal segments of the nephron [47]. Turtles also lack a tubular mechanism for altering renin release, but there is a well-developed renin angiotensin system in reptiles [13,48,49]. Seasonal variations in renin levels relate to the physiologic phase of the animals: active animals demonstrate high renal and plasma renin concentration, whereas lower values are obtained in hibernating animals [50].

The turtle urinary bladder is analogous to the collecting and distal tubules of the mammalian kidney and has been frequently used as an experimental model in renal physiology [51,52]. The epithelium of both the turtle bladder and the mammalian collecting duct may generate a steep gradient for H^+ ions between blood and urine. Secretion of H^+ into the urine is coupled with a basolateral efflux of HCO^-_3 that appears to be exchanged mainly against Cl^-. Knowledge of the large urinary bladders in terrestrial chelonids extends back to 1676, when the Parisian comparative anatomist Claude Perrault observed the extraordinary size of the urinary bladder in the Indian giant tortoise [53]. Under arid conditions, desert chelonids do not void but rather store urine in the bladder, where urine osmolality gradually rises. Potassium ions are precipitated with uric acid as urates, and the bladder can thus function both to store nitrogenous waste and K^+, as well as water that can be reabsorbed as needed. However, plasma osmolality gradually rises [54], mostly because of an increase in urea concentration. Urine is only voided following rain, when copious drinking restores bladder volume with hyposthenuric urine. In 1799, Townson observed that dehydrated freshwater turtles imbibed water by anal drinking [53]. More recent evidence indicates that this is not a method of hydration but rather enables the urinary bladder to supplement the respiratory exchange of oxygen and carbon dioxide [55,56].

Uricotely in birds and reptiles

In reptiles and birds, excretion of ammonia is achieved by first converting it to the amino acids glutamine (by means of glutamate), glycine, and aspartate for incorporation into the purine synthetic pathway. This pathway is much more energy expensive than the urea cycle of mammals, with the main advantage being the excretion of relatively insoluble nitrogen-rich uric acid, which is not reabsorbed from the cloaca in the adult or from the allantois in the avian embryo. In the egg, urate occurs as a crystalline anhydrous deposit in the allantois, not as a watery colloid gel as in the adult. This form permits efficient recycling of the transporting water and electrolytes and segregation of nitrogenous waste material. If urea, which is approximately 40,000 times more soluble than uric acid, were the primary nitrogenous waste product in avian and reptilian embryos, it would readily diffuse back into the blood in potentially toxic concentrations.

Birds do not lack any of the urea cycle enzymes; arginine, an essential amino acid in birds, may still be broken down by arginase to form urea. However, arginase is predominantly mitochondrial, not cytoplasmic as in mammals, and the highest concentrations occur in the kidney rather than the liver [57–59]. Avian arginase may be upregulated in birds fed high-protein diets and is inhibited by adenosine triphosphate, so when energy is not limited, urea is not produced [60,61]. In low ambient temperatures, some birds may conserve energy by increasing urea excretion and lowering uric acid excretion. Hummingbirds may excrete as much as 50% of waste nitrogen as ammonia, provided that water intake is not limited [62–64].

Most of the amino nitrogen and all of the purine nitrogen are thus broken down to uric acid (mainly by the liver), which at physiologic pH forms soluble salts (urates) with ammonia, Na^+, or K^+ ions. Uric acid is actively excreted by the tubular epithelial cells. Most birds excrete approximately 80% of renal nitrogen as dihydrates of uric acid in a supersaturated colloidal suspension, with the remainder excreted as urea or ammonium that enters the urine by glomerular filtration. Avian urine contains approximately

5 mg/mL of protein, which helps, at a metabolic expense, to maintain uric acid in colloidal suspension. This colloidal material does not contribute to the urine osmotic pressure, and the osmolality of the fluid component is largely due to Na^+, K^+, and Cl^-. Hence urine specific gravity measurements are not a reliable indicator of "urine concentration" in birds. Moreover, during times of dehydration, the urine may be refluxed from the cloaca into the colon for further water reabsorption.

Avian renal physiology

At first reckoning, avian kidneys appear to have a limited capacity to concentrate urine compared with those of mammals. Two types of nephron are seen, each composed of a glomerulus and a tubular system. Reptilian-type nephrons (RTNs) are the major type (60% to 90%) and lack a loop of Henle. Mammalian-type nephrons (MTNs) are less numerous. They possess a loop of Henle with thick and thin limbs and convoluted proximal and distal tubules and are arranged parallel to each other with their loops of Henle bound with the vasa recta into medullary cones to allow for counter-current exchange [65]. Thus, urine may be concentrated to some extent as it passes through the loop of Henle. By contrast, RTNs are not arranged in parallel, are confined to the renal cortex, and may only produce urine that is isotonic or hypotonic to plasma. However, all collecting ducts pass through a medullary cone in their path toward a ureteral branch, so that urine may be concentrated to some extent regardless of the nephron from which it originated. Desert-dwelling species generally have more MTNs (as many as 40%) than do birds with ready access to water. Many desert and water bird species also have a nasal gland that actively secretes salt. In these species the nasal gland is the major site of sodium ion secretion. Sea birds can survive by drinking salt water and may refuse to drink fresh water.

Individual avian nephrons have a low GFR compared with those of mammals, but the number of nephrons per kidney is much higher in birds, so that overall GFR is similar. Normally, more than 95% of the water of the original filtrate is reclaimed by tubular reabsorption. Variations from this pattern are achieved by regulation of GFR or reabsorption, both of which are controlled by AVT. AVT release from the neurohypophysis is stimulated greatly by a rise in ECF osmolality but only moderately by a decrease in ECF volume, such as one due to hemorrhage.

The avian nephron has a juxtaglomerular complex that, with salt and volume depletion, releases renin to stimulate the conversion of angiotensin I to angiotensin II. This process in turn promotes aldosterone-mediated Na^+ absorption, K^+ excretion, decreased GFR, and decreased urine flow. By contrast with mammals, the alternative release of aldosterone from the adrenal gland is not stimulated directly by elevations in blood K^+. Birds also produce atrial natriuretic peptide, which acts to increase Na^+ excretion.

The renal-portal system is a feature that birds share with reptiles. It consists of a ring of veins that receive blood from the pelvic limb, colon, and some of the structures in that region. The renal-portal ring is connected to the hepatic portal system, the caudal vena cava, and the intervertebral venous sinuses. The renal-portal system is separated from the systemic circulation by a valve that is innervated by adrenergic and cholinergic fibers. When the valve is closed, it prevents blood from directly entering the caudal vena cava, and therefore most of the blood enters the kidney or the hepatic portal system. Much of the blood flows into the kidneys, where it mixes with arterial blood from the efferent glomerular arteriole and participates in perfusion of the peritubular network, but it does not supply the glomeruli. As much as two thirds of the blood supply to the kidney comes via the renal portal system, and as much as 50% of renal blood flow may come from the ischiadic and external iliac veins combined.

In response to hypovolemia, shock, or sympathetic stimulation (ie, flight or fight response), the valve opens and blood is diverted into the vena cava. The plasma osmolality rises and stimulates AVT, which causes constriction of the afferent glomerular arterioles of the RTNs. Thus the nephrons with the least capacity to concentrate urine are no longer functioning. The shunting of blood to the peritubular network allows the kidney to continue excreting uric acid even though the GFR is greatly reduced. The MTNs, not all of which are functional during normal hydration, are recruited so that glomerular filtration occurs in those nephrons most capable of producing concentrated urine.

Dehydration usually does not notably elevate blood uric acid concentrations until GFR is decreased to the point where uric acid cannot be flushed through the nephron. The high-protein diet of carnivorous birds such as raptors and penguins causes them to have higher reference blood uric acid ranges, and postprandial elevations may also occur. Avian urine is usually acidic, owing to efficient reabsorption of bicarbonate.

The kidneys, intestinal tract, salt glands, skin, and respiratory tract all contribute to osmoregulation in birds. Except in ostriches (*Struthio camelus*) [66], urine that enters the urodeum may be refluxed into the coprodeum and colon for water reabsorption. This process may affect the specific gravity and electrolyte concentrations in expelled urine. In ostriches, no urine refluxes into the colon, and the coprodeum is not used for fecal storage. This pattern is facilitated by a well-developed recto-coprodeal sphincter. Instead, the coprodeum acts like a urinary bladder where final modification of urinary solutes occurs. Ostriches thus can pass two types of droppings, one containing feces and one containing solely urine.

Mammals

Unlike those in lower vertebrates, changes in mammalian GFR cannot be affected by varying the number of functional nephrons. For systemic blood pressures within all physiologic ranges, GFR is maintained at a constant value (approximately 120 mL/min). However, it may be regulated, primarily by neuroendocrine control of glomerular hydrostatic pressure (ie, blood pressure within the glomerular capillary bed) to maintain GFR in the face of altered systemic blood pressure or to respond to systemic changes in fluid or electrolyte balance, such as hemorrhage or dehydration.

The mammalian proximal convoluted tubule (PCT) is metabolically active, functioning as the "bulk transporter" to reabsorb approximately 70% of filtered ions and water. Water and solutes are reabsorbed in approximately equivalent amounts so that filtrate tonicity is unchanged. Concentrated urine is achieved by countercurrent mechanisms involving the loop of Henle (Fig. 2). Filtrate leaving the PCT passes into the thin limb of the loop of Henle where the tubular epithelium is permeable to water, but there is no active ion transport. In the ascending limb of the loop of Henle, Na^+, K^+, and Cl^- are actively pumped out of the filtrate and into the medullary interstitium. Urea is passively reabsorbed by facilitated (carrier-mediated) diffusion in the collecting duct [67] and contributes to the generation of a medullary concentration gradient. Vascular anatomy and blood flow are such that ions and urea are not effectively removed from the medulla, ensuring maintenance of this concentration gradient and hypertonic medullary interstitial fluid. Continued reabsorption of Na^+, K^+, and Cl^- ions in the distal convoluted tubule results in the production of hypotonic filtrate.

The distal convoluted tubule and collecting duct are selectively permeable to water, with the degree of water permeability regulated by the RAS, antidiuretic hormone (AVP), and natriuretic peptides, such as atrial natriuretic peptide (ANP). Angiotensin II acts to increase blood pressure by increasing aldosterone and AVP secretion, stimulating thirst and vasoconstrictive effects; it also acts directly on afferent and efferent glomerular vessels to preserve GFR (and hence urine output) in the face of decreased systemic blood pressure. Aldosterone increases the ability of principal cells of the distal nephron to reabsorb Na^+ from the filtrate. As a result, aldosterone concurrently increases K^+ excretion (because Na^+ reabsorption and K^+ excretion are inversely related) and increases water reabsorption (because water passively follows Na^+). AVP also increases water reabsorption from the distal nephron by upregulating the production and insertion of aquaporin channels into the apical membrane of principal cells, thereby increasing the permeability of the distal cells to water. With maximum permeability, water is reabsorbed until the filtrate is isosmotic with the medullary interstitium, at which point further water reabsorption cannot occur because a concentration gradient no longer exists. Water movement across epithelia is always passive, driven by changes in concentration—there is no such thing as a "water pump." Therefore, a mammal cannot produce urine that is more concentrated than the medullary interstitial fluid. ANP increases the number of open Na^+ channels in the apical membrane of principal cells, producing sodium diuresis and increased water loss and thereby opposing the changes induced by aldosterone and AVP.

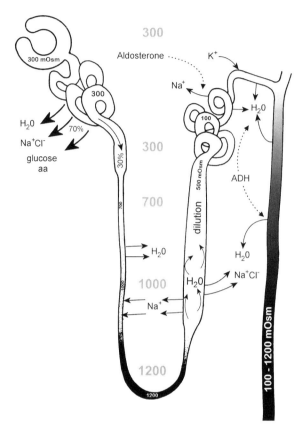

Fig. 2. High-pressure filtrate in the mammalian nephron passes into the proximal convoluted tubule, where most nutritionally important solutes (such as amino acids and glucose) and approximately 70% of filtered water and ions are reabsorbed in isosmotic amounts. The descending limb of the loop of Henle is permeable to water, but the flattened tubular epithelium lacks the cellular machinery for active reabsorption of solutes. Because of water loss, the filtrate becomes hypertonic relative to plasma in this part of the nephron. As the filtrate passes into the thick part of the ascending limb, solutes (particularly Na^+, K^+, and Cl^-) are actively reabsorbed, but the epithelium in this part of the nephron is impermeable to water. The selective removal of solutes thus dilutes the filtrate so that, by the commencement of the distal convoluted tubule (DCT), the filtrate is hypotonic relative to plasma. In situations of positive water balance (ie, needs to excrete excess water), the DCT and collecting duct will remain impermeable to water, and the filtrate will pass through the distal nephron with minimal further modification, being voided as dilute urine. Conversely, when the animal needs to conserve water, the water permeability of the DCT and collecting duct will be increased under the influence of increased circulating concentrations of antidiuretic hormone (ADH), so that water may freely leave the tubules. Water movement is driven by the concentration gradient achieved by high solute concentrations (primarily Na^+ and urea) in the medullary interstitium. Aldosterone acts to promote the active reabsorption of Na^+, which further increases water reabsorption. In this way, a smaller volume of more concentrated urine may be produced.

Fluid loss through the mammalian kidney may thus be minimized by concentrating renal filtrate to the degree that medullary interstitial fluid is concentrated. For humans, urine concentration cannot exceed 1200 to 1400 mOsm [68]. Greater concentrating ability is achieved in other species with fewer nephrons, increased proportion of juxtamedullary nephrons (which have longer loops of Henle than cortical nephrons), longer loops of Henle, increased medullary size, and longer renal papillae. For example, humans have approximately 17% juxtamedullary nephrons, whereas cats and dogs have approximately 100% of their nephrons located beside the medulla. The medullary/cortical ratio (M:C) is, in effect, a measure of the relative length of the loop of Henle for any species. In humans, the M:C is approximately five, whereas in cats it is eight, and in some desert animals it may approximate 20 [69]. This difference explains why felids can concentrate urine to 3300 mOsm, and some desert animals can produce urine of as much as 9000 mOsm [70,71].

Marine mammals such as cetaceans (whales and porpoises) cope in their hyperosmotic environment by markedly minimizing their respiratory and transcutaneous water losses and producing concentrated urine [72]. Water requirements are met through dietary intake and metabolic processes, primarily the oxidation of fat. Active or even incidental consumption of sea water is minimal in most species, with the exception of otters. In dolphins, the osmolality of urine is always higher than that of plasma and usually exceeds that of the surrounding ocean (see Table 1). Urine osmolalities are typically 1300 to 2000 mOsm for cetaceans [73] but may decrease under fasting conditions, when increased metabolic water is produced from fat catabolism [74,75]. Conversely, in pinnipeds (seals and walruses), urine concentration may be as great as 2500 mOsm [73]. Volume is reduced in fasting animals and urine concentration maintained or increased relative to feeding animals [76].

References

[1] Evans DH, Piermarini PM, Choe KP. The multifunctional fish gill: dominant site of gas exchange, osmoregulation, acid-base regulation, and excretion of nitrogenous waste. Physiol Rev 2005;85:97–177.

[2] Cameron JN, Heisler N. Ammonia transfer across fish gills: a review. In: Gilles R, editor. Circulation, respiration, and metabolism. Berlin: Springer Verlag; 1985. p. 91–100.

[3] Binstock L, Lecar H. Ammonium ion currents in the squid giant axon. J Gen Physiol 1969; 53(3):342–61.

[4] Cooper AJL, Plum F. Biochemistry and physiology of brain ammonia. Physiol Rev 1987;67: 440–519.

[5] Cameron JN, Batterton CV. Temperature and blood acid-base status in the blue crab, *Callinectes sapidus*. Respir Physiol 1978;35(2):101–10.

[6] Weihrauch D, Morris S, Towle DW. Ammonia excretion in aquatic and terrestrial crabs. J Exp Biol 2004;207:4491–504.

[7] Hrnjez BJ, Song JC, Prasad M, et al. Ammonia blockade of intestinal epithelial K^+ conductance. Am J Physiol 1999;277:521–32.

[8] Regnault M. Nitrogen excretion in marine and freshwater Crustacea. Biol Rev 1987;62:1–24.

[9] Athawale MS, Reddy SR. Storage excretion in the Indian apple snail, *Pila globosa* (Swainson), during aestivation. Indian J Exp Biol 2002;40:1304–6.

[10] Jezewska MM. The nephridial excretion of guanine, xanthine and uric acid in slugs (Limacidae) and snails (Helicidae). Acta Biochim Pol 1969;16:313–20.

[11] Goyffon M, Martoja R. Cytophysiological aspects of digestion and storage in the liver of a scorpion, *Androctonus australis* (Arachnida). Cell Tissue Res 1983;228:661–75.

[12] Taylor AA. Comparative physiology of the renin-angiotensin system. Fed Proc 1977;36:1776–80.

[13] Wilson JX. The renin-angiotensin system in nonmammalian vertebrates. Endocr Rev 1984;5: 45–61.

[14] Salzet M, Deloffre L, Breton C, et al. Review: the angiotensin system elements in invertebrates. Brain Res Rev 2001;36:35–45.

[15] Brauner CJ, Matey V, Wilson JM, et al. Transition in organ function during the evolution of air-breathing; insights from *Arapaima gigas*, an obligate air-breathing teleost from the Amazon. J Exp Biol 2004;207:1433–8.

[16] Nishimura H, Imai M, Ogawa M. Sodium chloride and water transport in the renal distal tubule of the rainbow trout. Am J Physiol 1983;244:247–54.

[17] Beyenbach KW. Kidneys sans glomeruli. Am J Physiol Renal Physiol 2004;286:811–27.

[18] Barimo JF, Steele SL, Wright PA, et al. Dogmas and controversies in the handling of nitrogenous wastes: ureotely and ammonia tolerance in early life stages of the gulf toadfish, *Opsanus beta*. J Exp Biol 2004;207:2011–20.

[19] Walsh PJ, Heitz MJ, Campbell CE, et al. Molecular characterization of a urea transporter in the gill of the gulf toadfish (*Opsanus beta*). J Exp Biol 2000;203:2357–64.

[20] Lim CK, Wong WP, Lee SM, et al. The ammonotelic African lungfish, *Protopterus dolloi*, increases the rate of urea synthesis and becomes ureotelic after feeding. J Comp Physiol [B] 2004;174:555–64.

[21] Hays RM, Levine SD, Myers JD, et al. Urea transport in the dogfish kidney. J Exp Zool 1977;199:309–16.

[22] Part P, Wright PA, Wood CM. Urea and water permeability in dogfish (*Squalus acanthias*) gills. Comp Biochem Physiol A Mol Integr Physiol 1998;119(1):117–23.

[23] Withers P, Hefter G, Pang TS. Role of urea and methylamines in buoyancy of elasmobranches. J Exp Biol 1994;188:175–89.

[24] Fines GA, Ballantyne JS, Wright PA. Active urea transport and an unusual basolateral membrane composition in the gills of a marine elasmobranch. Am J Physiol Regul Integr Comp Physiol 2001;280:16–24.

[25] Zeidel JD, Mathai JC, Campbell JD, et al. Selective permeability barrier to urea in shark rectal gland. Am J Physiol Renal Physiol 2005;289(1):F83–9.

[26] Morgan RL, Wright PA, Ballantyne JS. Urea transport in kidney brush-border membrane vesicles from an elasmobranch, *Raja erinacea*. J Exp Biol 2003;206:3293–302.

[27] Lee JA, Lee HA, Sadler PJ. Uraemia: is urea more important than we think? Lancet 1991; 338:1438–40.

[28] Haywood GP. A preliminary investigation into the roles played by the rectal gland and kidneys in the osmoregulation of the striped dogfish *Poroderma africanum*. J Exp Zool 1975;193: 167–75.

[29] Wendelaar Bonga SE. Endocrinology. In: Evans DH, editor. The physiology of fishes. Boca Raton (FL): CRC Press; 1993. p. 469–502.

[30] Amer S, Brown JA. Glomerular actions of arginine vasotocin in the *in situ* perfused trout kidney. Am J Physiol Regul Integr Comp Physiol 1995;269:775–80.

[31] Wells A, Anderson WG, Hazon N. Development of an in situ perfused kidney preparation for elasmobranch fish: action of arginine vasotocin. Am J Physiol Regul Integr Comp Physiol 2002;282:1636–42.

[32] Mahlmann S, Meyerhof W, Hausmann H, et al. Structure, function, and phylogeny of [Arg8]vasotocin receptors from teleost fish and toad. Proc Natl Acad Sci USA 1994;91(4): 1342–5.

[33] Guibbolini ME, Avella M. Neurohypophysial hormone regulation of Cl⁻ secretion: physi-ological evidence for V1-type receptors in sea bass gill respiratory cells in culture. J Endocri-nol 2003;176(1):111–9.

[34] Bond H, Winter MJ, Warne JM, et al. Plasma concentrations of arginine vasotocin and ur-otensin II are reduced following transfer of the euryhaline flounder (*Platichthys flesus*) from seawater to fresh water. Gen Comp Endocrinol 2002;125(1):113–20.

[35] Brown JA, Paley RK, Amer S, et al. Evidence for an intrarenal renin-angiotensin system in the rainbow trout, *Oncorhynchus mykiss*. Am J Physiol Regul Integr Comp Physiol 2000;278: 685–91.

[36] Hazon N, Tierney ML, Takei Y. Renin-angiotensin system in elasmobranch fish: a review. J Exp Zool 1999;284:526–34.

[37] Cobb CS, Williamson R, Brown JA. Angiotensin II–induced calcium signalling in isolated glomeruli from fish kidney (*Oncorhynchus mykiss*) and effects of losartan. Gen Comp Endo-crinol 1999;113(2):312–21.

[38] Wickramasinghe SN, Shiels S, Wickramasinghe PS. Immunoreactive erythropoietin in tele-osts, amphibians, reptiles, birds. Evidence that the teleost kidney is both an erythropoietic and erythropoietin-producing organ. Ann N Y Acad Sci 1994;718:366–70.

[39] Shiels A, Wickramasinghe SN. Expression of an erythropoietin-like gene in the trout. Br J Haematol 1995;90:219–21.

[40] Chou CF, Tohari S, Brenner S, et al. Erythropoietin gene from a teleost fish, *Fugu rubripes*. Blood 2004;104:1498–503.

[41] Shpun S, Katz U. Renal response of euryhaline toad (*Bufo viridis*) to acute immersion in tap water, NaCl, or urea solutions. Physiol Biochem Zool 1999;72:227–37.

[42] Peng G, Hillyard SD, Fu BM. A two-barrier compartment model for volume flow across amphibian skin. Am J Physiol Regul Integr Comp Physiol 2003;285:1384–94.

[43] Uchiyama M, Yoshizawa H. Nephron structure and immunohistochemical localization of ion pumps and aquaporins in the kidney of frogs inhabiting different environments. Symp Soc Exp Biol 2002;54:109–28.

[44] Bayomy MF, Shalan AG, Bradshaw SD, et al. Water content, body weight and acid muco-polysaccharides, hyaluronidase and beta-glucuronidase in response to aestivation in Austra-lian desert frogs. Comp Biochem Physiol A Mol Integr Physiol 2002;131:881–92.

[45] Hillyard SD. Behavioral, molecular and integrative mechanisms of amphibian osmoregula-tion. J Exp Zool 1999;283:662–74.

[46] Bradshaw SD, Bradshaw FJ. Arginine vasotocin: site and mode of action in the reptilian kid-ney. Gen Comp Endocrinol 2002;126:7–13.

[47] Stephens GA, Robertson FM. Renal responses to diuretics in the turtle. J Comp Physiol [B] 1985;155:387–93.

[48] Cho KW, Kim SZ, Kim SH, et al. Characterization of angiotensin I–converting enzyme ac-tivity in the freshwater turtle, *Amyda japonica*. Comp Biochem Physiol A 1987;87:645–8.

[49] Cipolle MD, Zehr JE. Characterization of the renin-angiotensin system in the turtle *Pseu-demys scripta*. Am J Physiol 1984;247:15–23.

[50] Vallarino M. Seasonal kidney and plasma renin concentration in *Testudo hermanni Gmelin*. Comp Biochem Physiol A 1984;79:529–31.

[51] Drenckhahn D, Oelmann M, Schaaf P, et al. Band 3 is the basolateral anion exchanger of dark epithelial cells of turtle urinary bladder. Am J Physiol 1987;252:570–4.

[52] Henke SE, Pence DB, Rue Manh T. Urinary bladders of freshwater turtles as a renal phys-iology model potentially biased by monogenean infections. Lab Anim Sci 1990;40:172–7.

[53] Jérgensen CB. Role of urinary and cloacal bladders in chelonian water economy: historical and comparative perspectives. Biol Rev 1998;73:347–66.

[54] Dantzler WH, Braun EJ. Comparative nephron function in reptiles, birds and mammals. Am J Physiol Regul Integr Comp Physiol 1980;239:197–213.

[55] King P, Heatvole H. Partitioning of aquatic oxygen uptake during different respiratory surfaces in a freely diving pleurodiran turtle, *Elseya latisternum*. Copeia 1994:802–6.

[56] King P, Heatvole H. Non-pulmonary respiratory surfaces of the chelid turtle *Elseya latister-num*. Herpetologica 1994;50:262–5.

[57] Traniello S, Barsacchi R, Magri E, et al. Molecular characteristics of chicken kidney argi-nase. Biochem J 1975;145:153–7.

[58] Kadowaki H, Israel HW, Nesheim MC. Intracellular localization of arginase in chick kidney. Biochim Biophys Acta 1976;437:158–65.

[59] Kadowaki H, Nesheim MC. An assay for arginase in chicken kidney. Comp Biochem Phys-iol B 1978;61:281–5.

[60] Ruiz-Feria CA, Kidd MT, Wideman RF Jr. Plasma levels of arginine, ornithine, and urea and growth performance of broilers fed supplemental L-arginine during cool temperature exposure. Poult Sci 2001;80:358–69.

[61] Koutsos EA, Smith J, Woods LW, et al. Adult cockatiels (*Nymphicus hollandicus*) metabol-ically adapt to high protein diets. J Nutr 2001;131:2014–20.

[62] Preest MR, Beuchat CA. Ammonia excretion by hummingbirds. Nature 1977;386:561–2.

[63] Roxburgh L, Pinshow B. Ammonotely in a passerine nectarivore: the influence of renal and post-renal modification on nitrogenous waste product excretion. J Exp Biol 2002;205:1735–45.

[64] McWhorter TJ, Powers DR, Martinez Del Rio C. Are hummingbirds facultatively ammo-notelic? Nitrogen excretion and requirements as a function of body size. Physiol Biochem Zool 2003;76:731–43.

[65] Goldstein DL, Skadhauge E. Renal and extrarenal regulation of body fluid composition. In: Whittow GC, editor. Sturkie's avian physiology. San Diego (CA): Academic Press; 1999. p. 265–98.

[66] Deeming DC. In: The ostrich: biology, production and health. Wallingford and Oxon (UK): CABI Publishing; 1999. p. 54–60.

[67] Sands JM. Regulation of renal urea transporters. J Am Soc Nephrol 1999;10:635–46.

[68] Guyton AC, Hall JE. In: Textbook of medical physiology. Philadelphia: WB Saunders; 2000. p. 264–345.

[69] Germann WJ, Stanfield CL. In: Germann WJ, Stanfield CL, editors. Principles of human physiology with interactive physiology. San Francisco (CA): Benjamin Cummings; 2004. p. 532–600.

[70] Schmidt-Nielsen K. In: Animal physiology: adaptation and environment. 4th edition. New York: Cambridge University Press; 1990. p. 458–75.

[71] Diaz GB, Ojeda RA, Dacar M. Water conservation in the South American desert mouse opossum, *Thylamyus pusilla* (*Didelphimporphia, Didelphidae*). Comp Biochem Physiol A Mol Integr Physiol 2001;130:323–30.

[72] Janech MG, Chen R, Klein J, et al. Molecular and functional characterization of a urea transporter from the kidney of a short-finned pilot whale. Am J Physiol Regul Integr Comp Physiol 2002;282:1490–500.

[73] Ortiz RM. Osmoregulation in marine mammals. J Exp Biol 2001;204:1831–44.

[74] Malvin RL, Rayner M. Renal function and blood chemistry in Cetacea. Am J Physiol 1968;214:187–91.

[75] Ridgeway SH. Homeostasis in the aquatic environment. In: Ridgeway SH, editor. Mammals of the sea: biology and medicine. Springfield (IL): Thomas; 1972. p. 590–747.

[76] Ortiz RM, Wade CE, Ortiz C, et al. Acutely elevated vasopressin increases circulating con-centrations of cortisol and aldosterone in fasting northern elephant seal (*Mirounga angustir-ostris*) pups. J Exp Biol 2003;206:2795–802.

[77] Evans DH. Osmotic and ionic regulation. In: Evans DH, editor. The physiology of fishes. Boca Raton (FL): CRC Press; 1993. p. 315–41.

[78] Hill RW, Wyse GA, Anderson M. Water and salt physiology of animals in their environ-ments. In: Animal physiology. Sunderland (MA): Sinauer Assoc; 2004. p. 685–719.

[79] Stinner JN, Hartzler LK. Effect of temperature on pH and electrolyte concentration in air-breathing ectotherms. J Exp Biol 2000;203(13):2065–74.

[80] Campbell TW. Blood biochemistry of lower vertebrates. In: 55th Annual Meeting of the American College of Veterinary Pathologists (ACVP) and 39th Annual Meeting of the American Society of Clinical Pathology (ASVCP). American College of Veterinary Pathologists and American Society for Veterinary Clinical Pathology. Middleton (WI): International Veterinary Information Service; 2004. p. 1104–245.
[81] Fudge A. Laboratory medicine, avian and exotic pets. Philadelphia: WB Saunders; 2000. 375–400.

ELSEVIER
SAUNDERS

Vet Clin Exot Anim 9 (2006) 33–67

VETERINARY
CLINICS
Exotic Animal Practice

Exotic Mammal Renal Disease: Causes and Clinical Presentation

Peter G. Fisher, DVM

*Pet Care Veterinary Hospital, 5201-A Virginia Beach Boulevard,
Virginia Beach, VA 23462, USA*

Renal disease is not uncommon in exotic mammals, with degenerative, infectious (bacterial, viral, parasitic), metabolic, nutritional, neoplastic, anatomic, and toxic causes all represented. This article discusses the clinical presentation for the various renal diseases affecting exotic mammals. Anatomic pathology at the gross and microscopic level is reviewed, as is disease pathophysiology unique to the species under discussion.

Ferrets

Renal pathology is not uncommon in the ferret, with many ferrets older than 4 years having various degrees of chronic interstitial nephritis [1]. A 1994 review of 61 cases submitted to the Registry of Veterinary Pathologists, Armed Forces Institute of Pathology, Washington, DC showed that the most prevalent causes of ferret renal pathology included acute nephritis (22%), renal cysts (15%), glomerulonephritis (14%), pyelonephritis (6%), glomerulosclerosis (4%), congestion (4%), and tubular atrophy (4%) [1]. Other causes of ferret renal pathology include Aleutian disease, toxic nephropathies, and renal disease associated with urinary tract calculi and neoplasia.

Aleutian disease

The Aleutian disease (AD) parvovirus is characterized by strains of variable virulence and immunogenicity that affect mink and ferrets. A fulminant, lethal infection in mink, the AD parvovirus is usually a chronic, latent infection in ferrets, which may cause clinical disease over a period of 1 to 2 years. It is suspected that transmission of the virus from ferret to ferret or mink to ferret occurs by aerosolization of or direct contact

---

E-mail address: peter.g.fisher@verizon.net

1094-9194/06/$ - see front matter © 2006 Elsevier Inc. All rights reserved.
doi:10.1016/j.cvex.2005.10.004   *vetexotic.theclinics.com*

with urine, saliva, blood, and feces or by contact with fomites. Although the parvovirus itself causes little or no harm to the ferret, the marked inflammatory response generated by the host results in production of a large number of antigen-antibody complexes. These circulate in the body and with time cause systemic vasculitis, most notably in the glomerular capillaries. As the disease progresses, a marked membranous glomerulonephritis and tubular interstitial nephritis result in eventual renal failure and death. In addition, a marked lymphocytic-plasmacytic response interferes with bone marrow hematopoiesis, and local accumulation of lymphocytes, plasma cells, and macrophages may result in multiple organ dysfunction and failure.

Manifestations of clinical disease are most likely determined by virus strain and host genotype and immune status [2]. In many ferrets the disease is manifested by chronic, progressive weight loss, lethargy, anemia, and melena, whereas other infected ferrets remain asymptomatic until shortly before death. Posterior paresis with progression to an ascending paralysis, tremors, seizures, and fecal and urinary incontinence may occur as a result of AD-related plasmacytic myelitis. Ferrets can survive this neurologic form of AD with supportive care; however, most eventually succumb to glomerulonephritis and kidney disease [3]. In end-stage disease, the marked hypergammaglobulinemia and vasculitis may result in anemia, thrombocytopenia, and altered platelet function, with subsequent petechial hemorrhage and clotting abnormalities. At the same time, a significant leukopenia predisposes the ferret to secondary bacterial infections.

Biopsy or necropsy specimens from infected ferrets (particularly the kidney, liver, spleen, mesenteric lymph nodes, and spinal cord) often yield a presumptive diagnosis. Gross lesions are seen only late in the course of disease, with splenomegaly and lymphadenopathy being most common. Enlarged, brown-tan kidneys may be present [3]. Several characteristic microscopic findings are seen in ferret AD. Prominent lymphocytic-plasmacytic infiltrates are seen in numerous organs, most prominently in the renal interstitium, hepatic portal areas, and the splenic red pulp. In most cases, there will be marked membranous glomerulonephritis and numerous ectatic (distended or stretched) protein-filled tubules [3]. Vasculitis may be seen in almost any organ.

Acute renal failure secondary to urethral obstruction

Acute renal failure and postrenal azotemia and uremia may occur in the ferret with urethral obstruction. The differential diagnosis for urethral obstruction includes urolithiasis or severe crystalluria, gross pyuria, urethral compression due to prostatomegaly or prostatic cysts (males) or other cystic paraurethral structures (males or females), and neoplasia (rare) [4]. As in other animals, urethral obstruction occurs more frequently in males than females. Ferrets with urethral obstruction will show various degrees of stranguria, dysuria, and pollakiuria. Depending on the duration and degree of obstruction, ferrets may show urinary incontinence or dribbling, with wet fur and excessive licking of the prepuce or perineum. Within 24 hours, ferrets will demonstrate behaviors consistent with abdominal pain, including depression, grinding of the teeth (bruxism), walking with an arched back, and vocalizing when urinating. Abdominal tenderness and a full, painful bladder will be evident on palpation. When the condition is secondary to prostatomegaly or periprostatic cysts, two or more firm-to-fluctuant masses will be palpable in the caudal abdomen. Radiographs should be taken to rule out urolithiasis. An adrenal hormone panel (Endocrinology Laboratory, University of Tennessee, Knoxville, Tennessee) should be submitted for ferrets with gross pyuria, prostatomegaly, periprostatic cysts, or other cystic paraurethral structures, because these conditions are common manifestations of primary adrenal disease. A complete blood count (CBC), biochemical analysis, urinalysis (by cystocentesis with a 25-gauge needle to prevent inadvertent rupture of the distended bladder), and urine culture and sensitivity should be performed.

Renal calculi

Bilateral or unilateral renal pelvis calculi have been reported in the ferret. Most are incidental findings on abdominal radiography and not associated with renal disease or azotemia. They may be associated with concurrent bladder or urethral calculi. Microscopic renal pathologic conditions associated with pelvic calculi include chronic diffuse glomerulonephritis, pyelonephritis, amyloidosis, focal glomerular fibrosis, and early tubular dilatation and necrosis [5]. Diagnosis is performed by radiography or ultrasonography.

The incidence of urolithiasis has declined as commercial diets for pet ferrets have improved nutritionally and gained acceptance among ferret owners. Current animal-based protein diets result in a more acidic urine than that associated with the plant protein–based diets previously in favor, decreasing the incidence of magnesium ammonium phosphate (struvite) uroliths.

Hydronephrosis

Hydronephrosis is an uncommon finding in the ferret. The author has seen two cases that resulted from inadvertent ligation of the ureter during ovariohysterectomy. Both ferrets presented for an obvious abdominal swelling that was most noticeable when in dorsal recumbency. Abdominal palpation revealed a midabdominal mass, approximately 6 by 10 cm, that was confirmed radiographically as a large radiopaque mass of uniform fluid density consistent with an enlarged kidney. Surgical exploration confirmed the diagnosis, and both cases were successfully treated by unilateral nephrectomy (Fig. 1). Presurgical biochemical renal parameters were normal, indicating a functional contralateral kidney.

Hydronephrosis in the ferret has also been reported secondary to obstruction with ureteral calculi [4]. A hydronephrotic kidney was also

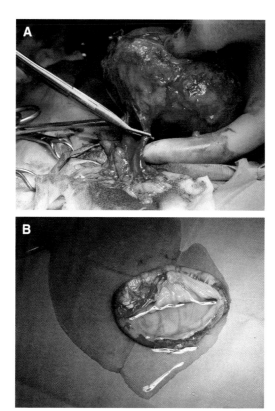

Fig. 1. (*A,B*) Surgical removal of a hydronephrotic kidney that resulted from inadvertent ligation of the ureter during ovario-hysterectomy in a female ferret. This ferret's blood chemistries
were normal owing to normal function of the opposite kidney.

reported in association with a carcinoma of undetermined origin involving
the renal pelvis [6]. In this 13-month-old spayed female ferret, the author
suspected a congenital atretic ureter or neoplastic stricture as cause for
the hydronephrosis, but histopathologic examination confirmed neither.

Chronic interstitial nephritis

Chronic interstitial nephritis is a common finding in ferrets; as in dogs
and cats, it is usually a progressive disease associated with aging. Early lesions may be seen as early as 2 years, and advanced cases resulting in renal
failure may occur as early as 4.5 years [7]. Progression of the pathologic condition may result in renal failure, but various degrees of chronic interstitial
nephritis are also commonly seen at necropsy of geriatric ferrets that have
died from other causes [4]. Clinical signs vary with severity of kidney pathology. Polydipsia and polyuria may be associated with early kidney failure,
with progression to anorexia, weight loss, and lethargy as chronic interstitial
nephritis and the uremia of chronic renal failure progress.

Kidneys with significant disease are generally pitted, and large focal depressions may be seen in the outer cortex as a result of scarring. Severely affected kidneys may be asymmetric with regard to size [7]. The pattern of microscopic changes associated with chronic interstitial nephritis in the ferret is unique [7]. At low magnification, there are linear bands of fibrosis that extend from the capsule inward. Periglomerular and glomerular fibrosis result in glomerulosclerosis. The interstitium is expanded by fibrous connective tissue, throughout which are scattered moderate numbers of lymphocytes and plasma cells. Tubules within these radiating streaks of fibrosis exhibit various degrees of atrophy. Pathologists who have little ferret tissue experience may be tempted to diagnose chronic infarction [7]. As the disease progresses, there is a diffuse glomerulosclerosis throughout the cortex, and fibrosis may progress so that large areas are devoid of functional glomeruli and tubules.

Toxic nephropathy

Ferrets are naturally curious and demonstrate a keen exploratory behavior. They are skillful at accessing storage areas where they may be exposed to a variety of toxins, including chemicals, cleaning agents, medications, and pest control products. Unsupervised ferrets can readily pry the tops off child-resistant bottles or chew through plastic containers to access potentially toxic medications. Iatrogenic drug toxicities are also common. Box 1 lists potential nephrotoxic agents reported by the American Society for the Prevention of Cruelty to Animals Animal Poison Control Center (ASPCA APCC) [8]. Because of the ferret's small size (<2 kg), severe toxicities may result

---

Box 1. Nephrotoxic agents

- Cadmium
- Cholecalciferol
- Diquat herbicides
- Ethylene glycol
- Mercury
- Nephrotoxic antibacterials: over-the-counter bacitracin, polymyxin-B, gentamicin, neomycin
- NSAIDs
- Oxalic acid
- Phenolics
- Rhubarb
- Zinc

Data from Richardson JA, Balabuszko RA. Managing ferret toxicosis. Exotic DVM Veterinary Magazine 2000;2(4):23–6.

from ingestion of small quantities of toxic agent. Pharmacologic agents that have nephrotoxic potential in dogs and cats (eg, nonsteroidal anti-inflammatory drugs [NSAIDs], aminoglycosides) may also adversely affect ferrets.

Ibuprofen toxicity

Ibuprofen has anti-inflammatory and analgesic properties and is classified as an NSAID. The pharmacokinetics and clearance rates of NSAIDs vary greatly among species and even among individuals in which they are used [9]. Ibuprofen toxicity in ferrets is not uncommon, with 46 cases of ibuprofen ingestion reported to the ASPCA APCC between January 1996 and March 2000 [10]. Data in this study indicate that clinical signs of ibuprofen toxicity in ferrets are more severe than those expected at similar doses in dogs. Death was reported in four ferrets, with the lowest dose associated with death being 20 mg/kg. Therefore, ingestion of just one 200-mg ibuprofen tablet is potentially fatal in many ferrets. Toxicosis by NSAIDs is related to the inhibition of prostaglandin formation [9]. Prostaglandins have a wide range of physiologic effects and are involved in regulation and protection of the gastrointestinal, renal, cardiovascular, and reproductive systems. In ibuprofen toxicosis, repair of gastrointestinal epithelium is inhibited, as is secretion of the protective mucous layer in the stomach and small intestine. Vasoconstriction is induced in the gastric mucosa, and renal blood flow, glomerular filtration, and tubular ion transport are inhibited [4]. The specific pathophysiology of ibuprofen in ferrets is relatively unknown.

Clinical signs of ibuprofen toxicosis include ataxia, tremors, depression, weakness, recumbency, coma, vomiting, diarrhea, melena, polydipsia, polyuria, and respiratory depression (Fig. 2). In the APCC study cited earlier, 13.7% of cases reported signs involving the urinary system (eg, polydipsia, polyuria, dysuria, and renal failure) [10]. In one fatal case of ferret ibuprofen toxicosis, histopathologic findings included rare granular casts in the renal tubules and medullary renal congestion [9]. Renal failure is a known common sequela to ibuprofen toxicity in the dog.

Zinc toxicity

Diffuse nephrosis and renal failure have been described in a colony of Australian ferrets where multiple deaths were attributed to accidental zinc toxicity [11]. Ferrets appear to be more susceptible than other species to excess dietary zinc [12]. In the case described, zinc poisoning occurred as a result of exposure to zinc-laden white powder from the galvanized-wire cages in which the ferrets were housed. With time and repeat cleaning, zinc-containing cage wire will form a "white rust" that easily contaminates exposed food items. Ferrets in this cage situation were fed raw meat pushed through the wire mesh or placed on the wire floor. Zinc toxicosis results in increased blood urea nitrogen (BUN) concentrations and proteinuria due to increased glomerular leakage and decreased tubular reabsorption by the damaged

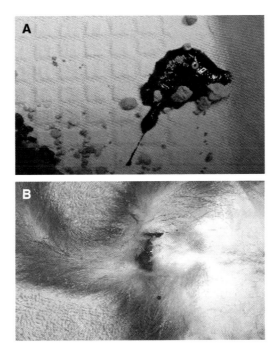

Fig. 2. (*A,B*) Melena is a common clinical sign associated with ibuprofen toxicity in the ferret. Renal failure as a result of reduced renal blood flow and inhibition of glomerular filtration and tubular ion transport is a common sequela to ibuprofen ingestion in the ferret.

tubules [12]. Experimentally induced zinc toxicosis caused diffuse cortical nephrosis characterized by dilatation of convoluted tubules with cellular debris, erythrocytes, and granular casts. Some glomeruli had dilated capsular spaces [12]. Zinc levels were highest in the kidneys (785 to 943 ppm, compared with levels of 110 to 120 ppm found in renal tissue of normal ferrets). Clinical signs reported with zinc toxicosis include anorexia, lethargy, anemia, melena, diarrhea, and icterus [4].

Other potential sources of accidental zinc poisoning include galvanized metal food and water bowls, zinc phosphide used as a rodenticide for anticoagulant resistant rats or as a grain fumigant to control insects, and zinc undecylenate–containing Desitin products (Pfizer, Morris Plains, NJ), calamine lotion, fertilizers, and suppositories. Many sources of zinc toxicosis seen in dogs or cats (plumbing nuts, pennies, Monopoly or jacks game pieces) are too large for a ferret to ingest.

Copper toxicity

Azotemia and hemoglobinuric nephrosis have been reported in sibling ferrets with copper toxicosis [13]. Both ferrets demonstrated central nervous system depression and lethargy. Copper toxicosis was diagnosed on the basis of liver histopathologic findings and high hepatic copper levels. Absence of illness in 11 other ferrets in the same environment fed the same diet suggested that the affected ferrets had an inherited defect in their ability to metabolize normal amounts of ingested copper.

Drug overdose

Veterinarians accustomed to working with dogs and cats must keep in mind the smaller size of ferrets and dose drugs appropriately based on an accurate patient weight in kilograms. A case of potential epinephrine and diphenhydramine overdose has been reported [14]. One milliliter of epinephrine of undetermined concentration followed by diphenhydramine at 10 times the recommended dosage was administered intramuscularly by a veterinarian for apparent vaccine-related anaphylaxis. The ferret developed progressive azotemia and died in spite of fluid diuresis, medical intervention, and supportive care. Necropsy findings included severe multifocal tubular necrosis, multifocal acute myocardial necrosis with contraction bands, and multifocal pulmonary edema. It was theorized that a high dose of epinephrine caused massive vasoconstriction, which led to decreased renal blood flow; the resulting anoxia predisposed to acute renal tubular necrosis [4]. The high dose of diphenhydramine potentiated the effects of epinephrine and enhanced the myocardial catecholamine toxicity.

Renal cysts

Renal cysts are not uncommon in ferrets, with the reported incidence as high as 10% to 15% of necropsied ferrets [15]. Renal cysts may be hereditary, developmental, or acquired [16]. Hereditary conditions include polycystic disease and several hereditary syndromes. Developmental conditions include renal dysplasia and renal cortical cysts. Acquired conditions include medullary cystic disease, postnecrotic cyst formation, endometriosis, and neoplasia [16]. The precise cause of cystic renal disease in the ferret is unknown, with one source presuming it is congenital in origin [17] and another citing speculation that chronic urinary tract infection leads to low-grade nephritis that predisposes the kidneys to cysts [7].

Most renal cysts do not cause clinical disease and are found incidentally during routine surgery, necropsy, or ultrasonography (as one or more hypoechoic areas). Most renal cysts have no effect on renal function. Cysts are usually present singly or in small numbers and are most commonly found in the cortices of one or both kidneys (Fig. 3). Cysts may range to as large as 1 cm in diameter; when viewed from the capsule surface, they are thin and fluid filled and bulge slightly [7]. On histopathologic examination of benign cysts, there may be little or no fibrosis surrounding the cyst, or the cyst may have a thick wall or fibrous connective tissue throughout, in which are scattered numerous atrophic glomeruli and tubules [7].

Polycystic kidney disease (PKD) has been reported in ferrets but is rare. Polycystic kidneys are grossly enlarged and may be palpable as a slightly

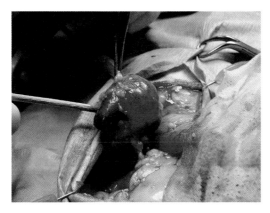

Fig. 3. This image demonstrates the gross in situ appearance of a ferret kidney with multiple cortical renal cysts. The large cyst seen here was associated with mild pericystic fibrosis and parenchymal atropy on histopathology. This ferret was not azotemic. The kidney cyst resulted in an obvious painful response on palpation; hence nephrectomy was recommended.

irregular, firm, oval mass or masses in the midabdomen (Fig. 4). Renal failure with uremic encephalopathy was suspected in one case of bilateral PKD where the cortex and medulla contained numerous fluid-filled cysts of various sizes [16]. Histologically, the cystic spaces were lined by cuboidal epithelium, with both fibrosis and areas of normal glomeruli and tubules in the intervening renal tissue [16].

Bilateral perinephric pseudocysts accompanied one case of PKD in an adult ferret [18]. In this case, survey abdominal radiographs showed two soft tissue radiopacities consistent with grossly enlarged kidneys. Follow-up

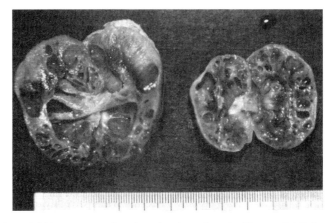

Fig. 4. Polycystic kidneys are grossly enlarged and may be palpable as a slightly irregular, firm, oval mass in the midabdomen. (*From* Dillberger JE. Polycystic kidneys in a ferret. J Am Vet Med Assoc 1985;186(1):74; with permission.)

abdominal ultrasound revealed bilateral perinephric pseudocysts and poly-cystic kidneys. The pseudocysts were drained by ultrasound-guided para-centesis, and the acquired fluid was distinguished from urine by measurement of creatinine concentration. The fluid rapidly recurred, but the ferret's conditions deteriorated, and euthanasia was performed before surgical resection of the renal capsule could be attempted.

Pyelonephritis

Pyelonephritis is uncommon in the ferret; when present, it is usually asso-ciated with an ascending bacterial urinary tract infection or septicemia. Necrotoxigenic *Escherichia coli* strains of hemolytic *E coli* have been cultured from the urine and kidneys of ferrets [19]. Urolithiasis and adrenal-associated prostatic disease are the most common causes of urinary tract infection in the author's practice, with *E coli* and *Staphylococcus aureus* being the most common causative agents. Severe, suppurative pyelonephritis progressing to end-stage chronic renal failure was reported in a ferret being treated for cutaneous epitheliotropic lymphoma [20]. In this case, the authors theorized that immunosuppression from long-term corticosteroid administration could have led to bacterial cystitis and subsequent pyelonephritis.

Clinical signs of pyelonephritis include pyrexia, lethargy, anorexia, and pain on palpation of the kidneys [4]. Chronic, untreated pyelonephritis may result in renal failure manifested clinically as profound anorexia and lethargy, with subsequent weight loss and declining condition.

Neoplasia

Urinary tract neoplasms are generally considered rare in ferrets. An ar-chive of 1525 ferret neoplasms compiled over a 10-year period (1990 to 2000) at the Armed Forces Institute of Pathology (Washington, DC) and Accupath (Potomac, Maryland), a commercial pathology laboratory, dem-onstrated six cases of primary or secondary neoplasia involving the kidneys [21]. Transitional cell carcinoma, the most commonly reported primary tu-mor of the ferret kidney, usually arises in the renal pelvis. As a result, this neoplasm may cause urine outflow obstruction and secondary hydronephro-sis or may completely efface all normal kidney tissue with neoplastic cells and fibrous tissue [6]. Renal cell carcinomas and adenomas have also been reported in the ferret [22]. These slow-growing tumors have little metastatic potential and are usually found unilaterally at surgery or necropsy (Fig. 5). Papillary tubular cystadenomas are benign and have only been reported once as an incidental finding [23]. The ferret kidney may also be the site of metastatic disease. In a retrospective study of malignant lymphoma in the ferret (1983 to 1990), stage IV lymphoma had invaded the kidneys in 8 of 18 ferrets [4]. Clinical signs of urinary tract neoplasia include hematuria, dysuria, incontinence, anorexia, lethargy, and weight loss. As with other neoplasms, biopsy and histopathologic evaluation of affected tissue are

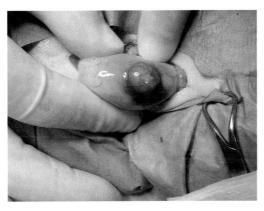

Fig. 5. This well-differentiated cystic papillary neoplasm (presumed adenoma) was found as an incidental finding during gastrointestinal biopsy surgery in a ferret with lymphoplasmacytic enteritis. This is an uncommon renal tumor in ferrets.

generally required for a definitive diagnosis. Ultrasound or other guided aspirates and cytologic evaluation may give a presumptive diagnosis.

Rabbit

Pathologic conditions of the kidney are not uncommon in the rabbit, with one review showing histologic lesions in 32.5% of 237 rabbits found dead or euthanized because of illness and in 25% of 77 apparently healthy adult rabbits [24]. Renal fibrosis, with or without dystrophic calcification, was the most common lesion observed in rabbits more than 10 months of age [24]. Lesions associated with an infectious process, such as renal abscesses, bacterial pyelitis, pyelonephritis, and nephritis, were the primary finding in rabbits 5 months of age or less [24]. Two cases of spontaneous amyloidosis, one associated with pyometritis and the other with renal calculi, were reported. Other causes of rabbit renal pathologic conditons include hypervitaminosis D, *Encephalitozoon cuniculi*, hydronephrosis, renal agenesis, renal cysts, and neoplasia.

Encephalitozoon cuniculi

Encephalitozoon cuniculi is a microsporidium, obligate intracellular protozoan parasite. Encephalitozoonosis appears to be a widespread disease in rabbits, with reports of infection found in 50% to 75% of conventional colonies [25]. Postnatal transmission occurs within 6 weeks from an infected dam or contact with other infected animals [25] and is the probable source of exposure in most pet rabbits. A spore, ingested or inhaled, is the infectious stage of *E cuniculi*. In the rabbit, infection of the host usually occurs by oral ingestion of spores from infected rabbit urine. The spore possesses a polar filament that it extrudes into host intestinal mucosa cells, injecting spore contents and initiating infection. Multiplication of the *E cuniculi* organism takes place in host alimentary cell vacuoles, with eventual cell rupture and spore invasion of the reticuloendothelial system and systemic circulation by infected macrophages. Initial target organs include those with high blood flow, such as the lungs, liver, and kidney [26]; infection of nervous tissue occurs later in the course of the disease. Organism multiplication occurs by ordinary fission or schizogony within vacuoles or pseudocysts (schizonts) found in reticuloendothelial cells of target organs. Spores eventually develop, and, with time, the pseudocyst becomes overcrowded and ruptures. Spores are spread to the urine by infected renal epithelial cells. Cell rupture is associated with a chronic inflammatory response and development of granulomatous lesions primarily in the kidney (Fig. 6) and central nervous system, although other organs, such as the heart and liver, may also be affected [27]. Serum antibody levels become detectable 3 to 4 weeks after infection, with maximum titers occurring 6 to 9 weeks after infection. Spores may be found in the urine 1 month after infection and are excreted in large numbers until 2 months post infection [28]. *E cuniculi* spores can survive outside the host for as long as 6 weeks at 72°F (22°C). Shedding of spores is essentially terminated by 3 months after infection [26]. Most immunocompetent rabbits develop chronic, subclinical infections in a balanced host–parasite relationship associated with granulomatous lesions primarily affecting the brain, kidney, or eyes.

The *E cuniculi* organisms spread to various organs; as antibodies develop, encapsulation occurs, limiting tissue damage and spore excretion. A healthy immune system prevents the organisms from multiplying, but the spores remain viable. Immunosuppression as a result of illness, stress, or aging may result in overt disease many years after initial infection. Antibodies contribute to resistance by inducing opsonization by macrophages and

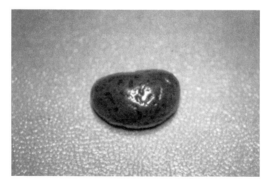

Fig. 6. This rabbit kidney demonstrates gross lesions associated with *Encephalitozoon cuniculi.* Irregular, pitted lesions of the renal cortex may occur with long-standing granulomatous inflammation caused by *E cuniculi*. Kidney lesions do not always impair renal function, and latent infections may occur. (*From* Harcourt-Brown FM. Textbook of rabbit medicine. Oxford (UK): Butterworth Heinemann; 2002. plate 31; with permission.)

complement-mediated killing [29]. Rabbits with encephalitozoonosis manifest a wide range of clinical signs, from absence of symptoms to death. The most commonly recognized neurologic sign is vestibular disease. In the eye, lens infection may lead to cataract development and phacouveitis secondary to lens rupture. *E cuniculi* is usually responsible for low-grade kidney disease in the rabbit. Histologically, early lesions show focal to segmental granulomatous interstitial nephritis. Lesions may be present at all levels of the renal tubule, and ovoid spores may be present within epithelial cells, in macrophages, in inflammatory foci, or free within collecting ducts [30]. In later stages, interstitial fibrosis is seen without evidence of the *E cuniculi* organism [26]. Kidney lesions do not always impair renal function, and latent infections can occur.

Polydipsia, polyuria, weight loss, and urinary incontinence with subsequent perineal scald are the most common signs associated with clinical renal infection. Biochemical evidence of kidney failure (elevated BUN and creatinine) may be seen in those rabbits manifesting more severe clinical signs (weight loss, anorexia).

A summary of serologic results includes rabbits with renal signs (polydipsia, polyuria, perineal scalding, weight loss, plus elevated BUN and creatinine) and antibodies against *E cuniculi* measured by ELISA. It shows that, in one study (United Kingdom, Harcourt-Brown) [27], 10 of 22 rabbits (45%) were serologically positive for *E cuniculi*; in another study (United States, Deeb) [29], 48 of 79 rabbits (61%) were serologically positive. These figures compare with a 37% and 49% positive antibody response in asymptomatic rabbits in the two studies, respectively.

Infections with *E cuniculi* have been reported in other exotic mammals, including mice, hamsters, and guinea pigs. *E cuniculi* has zoonotic potential, especially in immunocompromised humans.

Pyelonephritis/suppurative nephritis

Pyelonephritis in the rabbit may occur as the result of an ascending urinary tract infection or hematogenously during bacterial septicemia. Multifocal suppurative nephritis has been reported in a New Zealand White rabbit with a systemic *Staphylococcus aureus* infection [26]. *Pasteurella multocida* and *E coli* are other common organisms associated with rabbit pyelonephritis. Lesions and pathophysiology are similar to those described for mice.

Urolithiasis

Urolithiasis refers to the presence of calculi in the urinary system. The mineral composition of the most commonly diagnosed calculi includes calcium carbonate, calcium phosphate, and calcium oxalate. Rabbits have a unique calcium metabolism, in that nearly all dietary calcium is absorbed from the intestines and excess calcium is excreted in the urine. As a result, serum calcium levels fluctuate in proportion to dietary intake, and the excretion of calcium increases parallel to the amount of calcium ingested and varies directly with the serum calcium level [31]. Urine is the main excretory route of calcium in rabbits, and the high levels of urinary calcium precipitate into insoluble crystalline salts, resulting in cloudy urine. Rabbits on a high-calcium diet will produce the same volume of urine but with a proportionally higher calcium concentration. This process may result in the formation of "sludge," which over a period of weeks may progress by means of crystal aggregation to form a "muddy" stone, then a concretion, recognized in practice as a urolith or calculus [31]. Rabbits may have a combination of cystic, urethral, ureteral, or renal calculi (Fig. 7) [32]. Despite what is known about rabbit calcium metabolism, the exact cause or causes of stone formation are not understood and may relate to a combination of factors, including diet, genetics, anatomy, environment, and infection.

Clinical signs of urolithiasis may include lethargy, decreased appetite, weight loss, anuria, stranguria, hematuria, and a hunched posture and bruxism, indicating abdominal pain. Perineal soiling and subsequent scald may occur as a result of pollakiuria and incontinence. A turgid bladder is evident when urethral obstruction is present, and nephromegaly may be palpable when hydronephrosis occurs secondary to a ureterolith.

Calculus-related urethral obstruction may result in acute postrenal failure. Ureteral stone obstruction may lead to hydroureter and hydronephrosis with loss of kidney function. Renal calculi cause variable degrees of pelvic obstruction. Many renal calculi are bilateral or are present in conjunction with cystic calculi. Nephrolithiasis may be subclinical and found incidentally on abdominal radiographs (Fig. 8). With time, clinical signs of abdominal discomfort, hematuria, proteinuria, and isosthenuria may be seen. Eventually, chronic renal failure may ensue. An intravenous pyelogram may be performed to evaluate renal function.

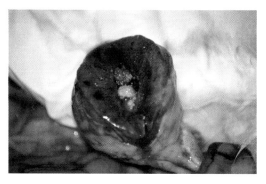

Fig. 7. This necropsy specimen is from a rabbit diagnosed with renal failure. The renal pelvis calculi seen here were found bilaterally. Histopathology and stone analysis were not performed in this case. (Courtesy of William Lewis, BVSC, MRCVS.)

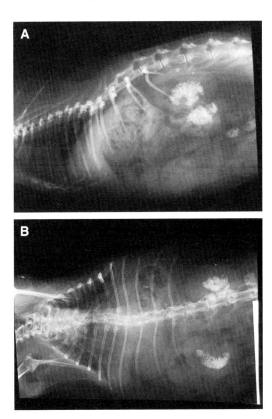

Fig. 8. (*A,B*) These radiographs show bilateral renal calculi in a female rabbit. Nephrolithiasis may be subclinical and found incidentally on abdominal radiographs. With time, clinical signs of abdominal discomfort, hematuria, proteinuria, and isosthenuria may be seen. Eventually, chronic renal failure may ensue.

Hypervitaminosis D

Rabbits are sensitive to vitamin D toxicosis, and levels as low as five times normal (>3000 mg/kg) may result in toxicity [33]. Adults are more sensitive than younger rabbits, and the toxicity induction period may vary from several weeks to several years depending on the individual's susceptibility and metabolism [34]. Pathologic changes consist of mineral deposition in various tissues, with arteries (especially the aorta) and kidneys being the most sensitive. Gross lesions in the kidneys consist of multifocal tan-to-gray areas located throughout the cortices [34]. Mineralization in the kidney occurs primarily in the basement membrane of the renal tubules and glomeruli, both of which may be surrounded by extensive interstitial fibrosis [34]. The exact pathophysiology of the soft tissue mineralization is unknown.

Clinical signs in rabbits suffering from vitamin D–related soft tissue mineralization are nonspecific and include anorexia, weight loss, dehydration, and infertility. Early clinical diagnosis is difficult, because clinical signs are nebulous. Because of the rabbit's normally high serum calcium level, the use of elevated serum calcium for detection of vitamin D toxicosis is of questionable value. In more advanced cases, radiographic evidence of soft tissue mineralization, especially of the aorta and kidneys, may be helpful in making the diagnosis.

Nephrotoxicosis

Gentamicin has been associated with nephrotoxicity owing to the direct effect of the drug on proximal tubular epithelium. Gentamicin also increases intracellular calcium levels in renal tubular cells and induces lesions of the apical membrane similar to those observed with calcium ionophore, indicating a possible role for calcium in the nephrotoxicity [35]. Vitamin B6 supplementation may help protect against gentamicin nephrotoxicity [36].

Dietary mycotoxins, aflatoxins and ochratoxins, have been associated with rabbit nephrotoxicity. Fungal growth and mycotoxin production may be seen in cereals and grains that are fed to rabbits, and production is influenced by moisture content greater than 13%, relative humidity greater than 70%, temperature greater than 55°F (13°C), and pH greater than 5 [37]. The toxicity of an individual mycotoxin relative to species depends on the breed, sex, and age of the animal, with old, young, immunocompromised, or physiologically stressed individuals being more susceptible to mycotoxicosis [37].

Use of intramuscular (IM) tiletamine/zolazepam (Fort Dodge Animal Health, Fort Dodge, Iowa) to induce anesthesia in rabbits has been associated with nephrotoxicity. Doses of 20 mg/kg or greater have resulted in azotemia as few as 3 days after injection [35]. Affected animals showed marked elevations in serum creatinine, BUN, and phosphorus. In rabbits given 32 mg/kg Telazol IM, urinalyses demonstrated hematuria, proteinuria, and granular casts 6 days after administration [38]. Histopathology of kidneys showed diffuse, moderate to severe nephrosis with various stages of degeneration and necrosis. Onset of clinical signs and severity of azotemia and nephrosis were dose related. Telazol is an injectable anesthetic composed of tiletamine and zolazepam in equal parts. Tiletamine, a dissociative anesthetic excreted by the kidneys, is the constituent responsible for the nephrotoxicity [35].

Neoplasia

Lymphosarcoma is reported as a common neoplastic condition in rabbits, with a higher incidence noted in juvenile and young adult domestic rabbits of less than 8 months of age. Anemia and azotemia may be seen clinically, and leukemia occasionally occurs. An autosomal recessive gene has been implicated as an important factor in susceptibility to the disease. Multiple organ involvement is common in both juvenile and adult spontaneous lymphosarcoma. Affected kidneys demonstrate multiple raised, pale, nodular masses, usually confined to the cortices. Different cell populations were observed in one case of multicentric, T cell–rich, B cell lymphoma reported in a 2.5-year-old Dutch dwarf rabbit [39].

Embryonal nephromas are commonly found in domestic rabbits, usually as an incidental finding at necropsy [40]. Embryonal nephromas of rabbits are typically benign and have been described in young and old rabbits, with the tumors generally becoming larger with age. Most tumors remain small (1 to 2 cm); however, tumors as large as 7 by 4 cm have been reported [40]. Secondary polycythemia of undetermined cause has been associated with rabbit embryonal nephromas. Diagnosis is usually made on abdominal palpation, radiographic or ultrasound examination, and ultimately biopsy of affected renal tissue. Unilateral nephrectomy is curative and allows for definitive diagnosis.

The Armed Forces Institute of Pathology has reported a case of spontaneous renal cell carcinoma in a 2-year-old New Zealand White rabbit.

Miscellaneous

Pet rabbits housed outdoors may develop a *Baylisascaris procyonis* infection from accidental contamination of feed by infective raccoon feces. Although this is primarily a disease of the central nervous system, kidney lesions (migrating larva tracts) may occur. Diagnosis is by identification of the parasite in tissue sections.

Fatty infiltration of the kidney has been reported in does with pregnancy toxemia. This disorder usually occurs during the last week of pregnancy in primaparous, obese animals on high planes of nutrition that suddenly become anorexic. Clinical pathologic abnormalities include ketosis, hypocalcemia, hyperphosphatemia, and fluctuating blood glucose levels. Fatty infiltration of the kidney with subsequent acute renal failure may also occur in conjunction with anorexia and development of hepatic lipidosis [30].

Multiple small subcapsular renal cysts are an inherited condition of rabbits. The cysts are either primitive ductules or of tubular origin, and the condition is similar to human renal cortical dysplasia [41]. An enlarged kidney may be palpated on physical examination or be detected on ultrasound examination or at necropsy. Renal cysts do not give rise to clinical signs or abnormalities in renal function or clinical pathology values.

Renal agenesis, or congenital absence of one kidney, has been reported as an autosomal recessive mutation in one colony of laboratory rabbits, and an increased incidence of this condition is reported in rabbits of the Havana breed [32]. The condition may be seen in both males and females, with males reporting concurrent absence of the ipsilateral testicle [32].

Masugi nephritis is an inflammatory nephritis seen in laboratory rabbits induced by continuous immunization with large doses of antigen. The condition results in elevations of BUN and creatinine [42].

Guinea pig

Urolithiasis

Like those of rabbits, guinea pig urinary tract calculi may be found in the urethra, bladder, ureter, or renal pelvis. Incidence is highest in middle-aged to older pigs, with females being more predisposed because the urethral orifice is close to the anus, allowing for contamination with fecal bacteria such as *E coli* and subsequent cystitis [43]. Calcium-based uroliths are most commonly found and include calcium carbonate, calcium phosphate, and calcium oxalate. Magnesium ammonium phosphate (struvite) calculi may be found as well [44]. Clinical signs vary with location and size of the calculus and may include dysuria, hematuria, pollakiuria, and anuria (vocalizing when attempting to urinate). Many pigs will show lethargy, have decreased appetites, and grind their teeth or have a hunched posture due to abdominal pain. Urethral calculi may result in obstruction and subsequent postrenal azotemia. Ureteral stones are especially painful and have been associated with hydroureter and hydronephrosis. Renal pelvic calculi may lead to obstructive nephritis and end-stage renal failure with time.

Diagnosis is based on suspicion with clinical signs and radiography or ultrasonography. Distal ureteral calculi are not uncommon in the guinea pig; hence multiple views are recommended when performing plain radiography to delineate anatomic location or locations of calculi. Ultrasonography has been used to diagnose a calcium carbonate ureterolith as a cause of ureteral obstruction and subsequent hydronephrosis in the guinea pig [45].

Renal parasitism

Renal coccidiosis from *Klosiella cobayae* has been reported in the guinea pig but is an uncommon finding. Clinical signs are normally absent, and the diagnosis is usually based on identification of the schizogonous stage in glomerular capillaries, or more commonly of schizonts or sporocysts in the cytoplasm of renal tubule epithelial cells [46]. The life cycle is direct and similar to that described in the mouse. A nonsuppurative inflammatory infiltrate of the renal tubules has also been noted [47]. Infected animals clear when housed in wire-floored cages, a measure that prevents contact with infective urine. Sulfadimethoxine and trimethoprim-sulfa may also be effective in treating this renal parasitism [48].

Cytomegalovirus infection

Cytomegaloviruses (CMV) are species-specific members of the Herpesvirus family. Naturally occurring CMV infections rarely cause clinical disease in the guinea pig and may persist in the host as an inapparent or latent infection for years [46]. Focal destructive lesions with large intranuclear and cytoplasmic inclusion bodies have been observed in the kidney [46].

Spontaneous generalized CMV infection with mortality seldom occurs, and lesions are usually regarded as incidental findings at necropsy.

Renal pathologic conditions associated with metabolic disease

Renal lesions may be seen secondary to metabolic disease in guinea pigs. In advanced cases of diabetes mellitus, histopathologic renal lesions include thickening of the basement membranes of the glomerular tufts, with or without sclerosis, and scarring of Bowman's capsule [46]. Pregnancy toxemia is most commonly seen in obese sows during the final 2 weeks of gestation. Characterized by anorexia and severe depression, pregnancy toxemia is precipitated by reduced nutritional intake and the mobilization of fat as a source of energy. Microscopic fatty change may be seen in the kidneys, liver, and adrenal glands. Subsequent circulatory collapse may result in subcapsular hemorrhages in the kidneys and necrosis of the proximal tubular cells.

Metastatic calcification

Metastatic calcification occurs most often in guinea pigs older than 1 year and is not uncommon. Clinical signs vary with severity of mineral deposition and organs affected. In mild cases, pigs are asymptomatic. Muscle stiffness and unthriftiness occur with mineral deposition in the soft tissues around the ribs and elbows. More widespread mineralization of tissues, including the kidneys, may occur. Metastatic calcification has been associated with feeding guinea pigs commercial rabbit pellets [47]. Dietary factors such as low magnesium and high phosphorus intake have also been incriminated in this syndrome [46]. Multifocal areas of mineralization in the renal pelvis with dilated cortical tubules have been reported in association with *Streptobacillus moniloformis* granulomatous pneumonia in the guinea pig [49].

Renal cysts

Renal cysts are uncommon and usually incidental findings on necropsy or surgery. The cysts may be single or multiple and may occur within the cortex or at the corticomedullary junction of one or both kidneys. It is speculated that the cysts arise from gradual distention of the nephron (obstruction by exudates or fibrous tissue), although the cause is seldom determined [47]. Definitive diagnosis is made by histopathology.

Segmental nephrosclerosis

Irregular pitting and a granular appearance to the renal cortices are common renal changes found at necropsy of guinea pigs more than 1 year old. The exact pathogenesis of this segmental interstitial renal scarring is unknown, but proposed theories have included association with an unusually high-protein diet, autoimmune disease, infectious diseases, and vascular disease resulting in focal ischemia and fibrosis [46]. On microscopic examination, there is segmented to diffuse interstitial fibrosis, with distortion and obliteration of the normal architecture [46]. Most glomeruli, however, are normal histologically. The disease is frequently considered an incidental finding, but advanced cases of nephrosclerosis may result in renal compromise, with elevated BUN and serum creatinine levels, isosthenuria, and non-regenerative anemia all reported.

Infectious disease

A multifocal necropurulent nephritis has been associated with a guinea pig yersiniosis [50]. Subacute interstitial nephritis has been reported in gnotobiotically reared guinea pigs that were seropositive for *Encephalitozoon cuniculi* [51].

Rat

Chronic progressive nephrosis

Chronic progressive nephrosis (CPN) is a common life-limiting disease in the older rat. Also known as progressive glomerulonephrosis, old rat nephropathy, or glomerulosclerosis, CPN is associated with aging and may affect 75% or more of susceptible strains. Clinical signs associated with the disease include significant proteinuria, isosthenuria, weight loss, and, as the disease progresses, elevated plasma creatinine levels consistent with renal insufficiency [52]. A number of predisposing factors may play a role in the development of CPN. They include (1) sex: male rats develop a more severe form of the disease and usually earlier in life than females; (2) age: lesions are more severe in rats older than 12 months; (3) diet: high-protein diets designed for superior body growth result in earlier onset of more severe disease; (4) strain: a significantly higher incidence of CPN is seen in the Sprague-Dawley rat; and (5) endocrine: prolactin levels are suspected of contributing to more severe disease [52].

Grossly affected kidneys are variably enlarged and pale, with pitted and irregular renal cortices that often contain pinpoint cysts (Fig. 9) [53]. On cut surface, there may be irregularities and linear streaks in the cortex and medulla, with various degrees of brown pigment [52]. The marked proteinuria associated with CPN is the result of microscopic changes consistent with a chronic glomerulopathy. Glomerular changes vary from minimal thickening of the basement membranes to marked thickening of glomerular tufts with segmental sclerosis and adhesions to Bowman's capsule [52]. The convoluted tubules are frequently dilated and lined by flattened or sclerotic epithelial cells with various degrees of basement membrane thickening, interstitial fibrosis, and mononuclear cell infiltration [52]. Renal secondary hyperparathyroidism, with mineralized deposits in kidney, gastric mucosa, lung, and the media of larger arteries, may occur in advanced cases [52].

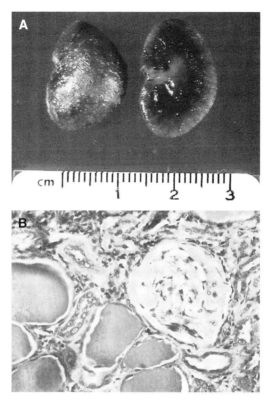

Fig. 9. (*A,B*) This rat died of CPN. (*From* Donnelly TM. Diseases of small rodents. In: Quesenberry KE, Carpenter JW, editors. Ferrets, rabbits and rodents: clinical medicine and surgery. 2nd edition. Philadelphia: WB Saunders; 2003. p. 307; with permission.)

Nephrocalcinosis

Nephrocalcinosis is observed on occasion in laboratory rats, including animals on regular commercial diets [52]. The disease is more common in females and may be found in animals as young as 7 weeks. Prevalence is as high as 50% in some strains of rat, with the F 344 and Wistar strains being most commonly affected. The disease may be the result of a number of dietary factors, including magnesium deficiency, elevated dietary phosphorus or calcium, and diet preparations with a low calcium-to-phosphorus ratio. Blood estrogen levels may also play a role, because the disease may be prevented by ovariectomy and is induced in castrated male and female rats by estrogen administration [44].

Renal lesions are characterized by the deposition of calcium phosphates in the interstitium of the corticomedullary junction, with intratubular aggregations in the same region [52]. Intraluminal concretions are usually associated with atrophy and loss of tubular cells but may also be associated with tubular dilatation and hyperplasia [44]. Thickening of basement membranes with deposition of collagen occasionally produces a chronic granulomatous inflammatory reaction [44]. Definitive diagnosis is based on histopathology. Onset of dietarily induced nephrocalcinosis may be rapid and is usually irreversible. Morbidity varies from slight to none to significant, depending on the progression of disease and severity of lesions.

Parasites

Klosiella hydromyos has been identified in Australian water rats (*Hydromys chrysogestes*), and an unnamed *Klosiella* sp has been identified in albino laboratory rats and the wild *Rattus rattus* [44]. Pathophysiology is similar to that of klosiellosis in mice. The bladder threadworm *Trichosomoides crassicauda* may be seen in *R rattus,* with as many as 80% of adult rats infected in some commercial colonies. The adult parasite normally resides in the bladder but may ascend to the kidney, causing acute or chronic renal pyelitis associated with hyperplastic lesions and urolith formation [44]. Ivermectin will treat bladder threadworm; prevention involves improved husbandry and sanitation.

Hydronephrosis

Hydronephrosis is often reported as an incidental necropsy finding in the rat and occurs in various strains. In some strains (Brown Norway, Gunn, Spague-Dawley), there is a hereditary basis for the disorder. Hydronephrosis may also be associated with ureteral calculi. The prevalence is higher in male rats. Hydronephrosis may be unilateral or bilateral and vary from mild to severe dilatation of the renal pelvis with associated excavation of the renal medulla. In severely affected animals, the kidney consists of a fluid-filled sac containing serous fluid [52]. The gross differential diagnosis includes pyelonephritis, renal papillary necrosis, and polycystic kidneys. If the condition is unilateral, diagnostic suspicion may be made on abdominal palpation of an enlarged kidney confirmed by radiography or ultrasonography. Clinical disease only occurs in severe bilateral hydronephrosis.

Suppurative pyelonephritis/nephritis

Rats can have bacterial infections anywhere in the urinary tract. Incidence is higher in older male rats. Suppurative renal lesions may be the result of an ascending bacterial cystitis or prostatitis; however, systemic hematogenous pyelonephritis has been discussed. A variety of bacteria have been cultured from infected kidneys, including *Pseudomonas* spp, *Proteus* spp, *E coli,* and *Klebsiella* spp [52]. Diagnosis is often made on history or clinical signs consistent with cystitis, urinary culture and sensitivity, and abdominal radiography or ultrasonography. Treatment includes fluid diuresis and long-term (4- to 6-week) antibiotic therapy based on results of bacterial culture and antimicrobial sensitivity.

Neoplasia

Neoplasia has been studied extensively, because rats serve as animal models of human disease. Many rats do not show signs of clinical disease or renal failure until they have advanced disease, and the prognosis is generally poor for affected animals. Renal cortical epithelial carcinoma, adenoma, and adenocarcinoma have all been reported, as well as renal pelvic epithelial papilloma, transitional cell carcinoma, and squamous cell carcinoma [44]. Metastatic or primary connective tissue tumors involving the kidney include lipoma, liposarcoma, fibrosarcoma, hemangiosarcoma, and leiomyosarcoma [44]. Diagnosis is usually made with a combination of history, physical examination, serum chemistries, urinalysis, and radiography/ultrasonagraphy. If the neoplasia is unilateral and localized, surgical resection may be attempted.

Miscellaneous

- Urinary calculi have been reported in the renal pelvis of the rat [52]. The composition of calculi is variable, with struvite (magnesium ammonium phosphate) most commonly seen.
- Male rats have been diagnosed with urinary proteinaceous plugs that may attain a large size and occlude the bladder lumen, leading to acute postrenal failure [44]. Treatment involves cystotomy to relieve the blockage, followed by fluid diuresis and supportive care.
- Renal papillary hyperplasia has been reported in hybrid Lewis and Brown Norway rats. Lesions are more common in males; they are generally confined to the renal papilli and consist of focal urothelial proliferative changes with hemorrhage and stromal necrosis [51]. Some rats have concurrent unilateral or bilateral hydronephrosis.
- Multifocal suppurative renal lesions have been associated with *Corynebacterium kutscheri* infection. This gram-positive bacillus is frequently harbored as an inapparant infection but may cause disease with a concomitant viral infection, nutritional deficiency, or state of immunosuppression [52].
- Polycystic kidney disease has been reported in the rat. The disease is usually spontaneous and transmitted as an autosomal recessive, monogenic disorder [54]. Many cases progress to massive cyst formation and renal insufficiency. Diagnosis is generally made on physical examination, clinical signs, serum chemistries and urinalysis, and radiography/ultrasonography.

Mouse

Pyelonephritis and nephritis

Grossly, bacterial lesions of the kidney generally have a focal distribution; however, they may be disseminated throughout the organ. Acute lesions vary from whitish, pale foci or nodules to, in severe cases, enlarged, swollen kidneys that are whitish to red [55]. Chronic cases are infrequently seen and are characterized grossly by irregular-shaped scars and depressions that extend from the kidney surface to the renal pelvis [55]. The microscopic appearance of the lesion depends on the micro-organism involved, the severity and age of the lesion, and whether the lesion is hematogenous or ascending in origin [55]. Nephritis of hematogenous origin generally involves the renal cortex and in the early stages may be centered in the glomeruli [55]. As the lesion increases in severity, it extends into the adjacent tubules, where abscessation may occur. Further extension down the tubules may result in pyelonephritis. Ascending infections always involve the renal pelvis and may secondarily spread to the renal cortex in an irregular fashion. Both types, ascending and hematogenous infections, are characterized by extensive infiltration with neutrophils that may result in complete destruction of the renal architecture [55]. Organisms that elicit a granulomatous reaction generally produce more focal lesions, with histiocytes as the predominant infiltrating cell [55].

Proteus mirabilis–induced suppurative nephritis and *Pseudomonas aeruginosa*–induced pyelonephritis have both been reported sporadically in mice [55]. Pyelonephritis as a result of an ascending *Streptococcus agalactiae* infection and subsequent septicemia has also been reported in mice, with bacterial colonies found in glomerular tufts and vessels within the kidney medulla [56]. Renal amyloidosis is a common secondary histologic feature of chronic pyelonephritis [57].

The mouse kidney is also a frequent site for lesions produced by *Corynebacterium kutscheri*. Stress-initiated disease is associated with the activation of latent infections [55]. Lesions in the kidney appear to be hematogenous in origin, because bacterial thrombi may be noted in glomerular capillaries that produce a liquefactive necrosis surrounded by a zone of neutrophils. The lesion generally progresses to large abscesses and may extend down the tubules in a linear pattern. Smears of the lesion may reveal a gram-positive, rod-shaped organism.

Diagnosis of pyelonephritis is ideally based on culture results accompanied by the histologic demonstration of the organisms within the lesions. Smears from fresh lesions stained for bacteria will often permit a rapid, presumptive diagnosis.

Leptospirosis

Mice may be infected with a number of *Leptospira* serotypes, but *L ballum* is particularly common [56]. Rodents do not become clinically ill when naturally infected and may shed organisms in their urine throughout life [56]. Lesions are generally absent in naturally acquired infection, but experimental inoculation of mice with *L interogans* serovar *icterohaemorrhagiae* results in renal tubular necrosis and interstitial nephritis. Diagnosis is made by kidney or urine culture and serology. *Leptospirosis* is zoonotic [44], and infected humans may develop flu-like symptoms after handling asymptomatic infected mice.

Parasitic infections

Renal coccidiosis due to *Klossiella muris* is rarely observed in laboratory mice but is quite common in wild mice [56]. *Klossiella* was also described in a breeding colony of Egyptian spiny mice (*Acomys cahirinus*) [58]. The genus *Klossiella* are protozoa belonging to the order Eucoccidiorida, which includes many parasitic organisms referred to as coccidia. *Klossiella* organisms localize in the convoluted tubules of the kidneys and are generally considered an incidental finding on necropsy.

Rodents acquire the infection by ingestion of sporulated sporocysts, each containing approximately 30 to 35 sporozoites. Released sporozoites then enter the blood, are transported throughout the body, and pass into the endothelial cells lining the kidney arterioles and glomerular capillaries, where schizogony takes place. Infection is usually nonpathogenic and asymptomatic; however, heavy infections may involve focal tubular degeneration and necrosis, with degenerative changes and hypertrophy also seen [59]. Gross lesions (gray discolored foci visible over the renal cortical surface) are only present in heavily parasitized animals [44]. On the cut surface, the lesions are in the corticomedullary region. Microscopically, the lesions demonstrate foci of necrosis characterized by a chronic granulomatous lymphocytic infiltrate and lymphocytic perivascular cuffing.

Diagnosis is usually made on renal histopathology performed during routine necropsy. If infection is found in a rodent colony, treatment with coccidiostatic preparations is advised, because *Klossiella muris* may impair the metabolism of mice [60]. Prevention and control of *Klossiella muris* in laboratory rodents involves proper sanitation to prevent spread by urine. Management techniques such as wild mouse control, cesarean delivery with separation from dam, and housing rodents in hanging cages that control contact with bedding and feces may help to prevent re-infection.

Diabetic nephropathy

Diabetic nephropathy is seen in the db/db laboratory mouse in which cell hypertrophy of the different glomerular cell compartments results in renal hypertrophy, thickened glomerular capillary basement membranes, and mesangial matrix expansion with subsequent albuminuria [61]. The db/db mouse serves as a model for human diabetic nephropathy.

Hereditary kidney disease

Hereditary kidney disease is not uncommon in laboratory mice. The ICR-derived glomerulonephritis mouse is an inbred mouse strain that develops proteinuria, hypoproteinemia, and anemia and is considered a good model for human idiopathic nephrotic syndrome [62]. Mice that are homozygous for the kidney disease gene on chromosome 10 spontaneously develop a progressive and fatal interstitial nephritis; the disease phenotype is similar to that of human juvenile nephronophthisis [63].

Chronic glomerulonephritis/glomerulopathy

Renal lesions are common in certain strains of older mice. Deposition of antigen-antibody complexes on glomerular basement membranes may occur as the result of persistent retroviral and bacterial infections [56]. In advanced cases, marked pitting of cortical surfaces may be seen on the gross level. Microscopic changes include proliferation of mesangial cells and thickening of glomerular basement membranes due to deposition of periodic acid–Schiff–positive material that does not stain for amyloid [56]. Focal to diffuse mononuclear cell infiltration and various degrees of interstitial fibrosis are other microscopic changes that commonly occur. Renal insufficiency with proteinuria and abnormalities in blood chemistries are seen in advanced cases of glomerulopathy.

Interstitial nephritis

The causes of tubulointerstitial disease in mice are similar to those in other species and include sequelae to bacterial infections, lymphocytic choriomeningitis virus, and chemically induced disease [56]. Depending on the duration and extent of the disease process, renal lesions may be mild and an incidental finding, or they may be of sufficient magnitude to contribute to the animal's demise. On microscopic examination, lesions may vary from discrete aggregations of mononuclear cells in perivascular regions of the renal cortex, to diffuse segmental involvement with distortion and loss of tubules, to obliteration of normal renal architecture in advanced cases [56].

Hydronephrosis

Hydronephrosis, unilateral or bilateral, is a common finding in the mouse. Hydronephrosis may occur in certain strains or lines of mice or be secondary to urinary obstruction or pyelonephritis [56]. Urinary obstruction is more common in male mice as a result of proteinaceous plugs or calculi that block the neck of the bladder and proximal urethra. In chronic cases of partial obstruction, dribbling of urine and perineal/preputial scald and dermatitis may be seen.

Amyloidosis

Primary spontaneous amyloidosis may be seen as an aging process in certain strains of laboratory or wild mice, or amyloidosis may appear secondary to chronic inflammatory disease or acariasis. Stress (crowding, fighting) and ectoparasitism may affect the prevalence of spontaneous amyloidosis [56].

Amyloid is a chemically diverse family of insoluble proteins that are deposited in tissues in a biophysical polymerized conformation known as the beta-pleated sheet. It is not known why these native biologic products are not catabolized. Amyloid deposition occurs in renal glomeruli, renal interstitium, myocardium, aorta, adrenal cortex, thyroid gland, and other tissues. Mice with amyloid deposition in the renal medullary interstitium can develop papillary necrosis. Amyloidosis is a progressive disease. Once a glomerulus has been irreversibly damaged by amyloidosis, the entire nephron becomes nonfunctional and is replaced by scar tissue. As more and more nephrons become involved, glomerular filtration decreases, and chronic renal failure ensues. It is a major life-limiting disease in aging mice that is confirmed by the typical appearance of amyloid and its staining characteristics on histology.

Hamster

A number of different genera and species of hamster are kept as pets or used as laboratory animals. The most common species seen in pet practice include the Syrian or golden hamster (*Mesocricetus auratus*), the Siberian or dwarf hamster (*Phodopus sungorus*), and the Chinese hamster (*Cricetulus griseus*). The information on hamster renal disease presented here concerns primarily the Syrian hamster; generalizations should be avoided, because the various hamsters kept as pets represent different, distantly related genera.

Amyloidosis

Amyloidosis is a common geriatric disease in Syrian hamsters for which the precise pathogenesis is poorly understood. Amyloid is an insoluble pathologic proteinaceous substance, deposited between cells in various tissues and organs of the body. Systemic amyloidosis may be classified as primary (amyloid light chain), secondary (amyloid associated), or familial [47]. Secondary amyloidosis is more commonly described in animals and may be a reaction to diverse inflammatory stimuli.

Amyloidosis occurs earlier in females and more frequently in certain strains, with prevalence as high as 36% in one report [64] and as high as 88% in another colony of hamsters more than 18 months of age [65]. Nephrotic syndrome is frequently associated with renal amyloidosis in hamsters and reflects the amyloid deposition along glomerular basement membranes. The resulting glomerulopathy causes severe loss of protein through the urine and a subsequent nephrotic syndrome characterized by malaise, edema (ascites, hydrothorax, anasarca), hypoalbuminemia, hyperlipidemia, and eventual cachexia (Fig. 10A, B) [66]. Kidneys may be grossly pale with atrophy and pitting of the cortical surface. On microscopic examination, the liver, kidneys, and adrenal glands are most frequently involved [67]. Histopathologic changes seen in one colony of Syrian hamsters consisted of extensive amyloid deposition in glomerular tufts, peritubular areas, and interstitial

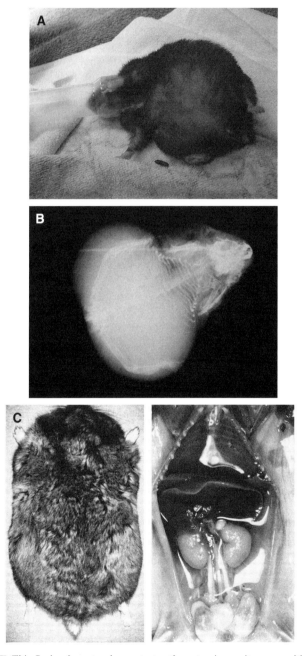

Fig. 10. (*A,B*) This Syrian hamster demonstrates the extensive ascites seen with hamster ne-phrotic syndrome. (*C*) The necropsy specimen shows the characteristic hydrothorax, ascites, and granular appearance to the kidneys. (Part *C from* Murphy JC, Fox JG, Niemi SM. Nephrotic syndrome associated with renal amyloidosis in a colony of Syrian hamsters. J Am Vet Med Assoc 1984;185(11):1360; with permission.)

tissues accompanied by numerous dilated tubules containing proteinaceous casts [66]. Extensive amyloid deposits were also seen in the liver, spleen, and adrenal glands of affected hamsters in this report.

Diagnosis is based on serum and urine analysis and clinical signs, which include ascites or subcutaneous edema concentrated in the ventral half of the body, hydrothorax, anorexia, and weight loss (Fig. 10C). Severe proteinuria and hypoalbuminemia are characteristic of significant glomerular disease, with elevations in BUN and creatinine occurring as renal failure ensues. Nephrotic syndrome is characterized by hyperlipidemia (elevated cholesterol and triglycerides), along with proteinuria, hypoalbuminemia, and clinical edema.

Arteriolar nephrosclerosis (hamster glomerulonephropathy)

Syrian hamsters may develop spontaneous renal lesions that resemble those of arteriolar nephrosclerosis in man [68]. This degenerative renal disease is associated with aging and is more frequent in females [67]. The causation and pathogenesis of the disease are poorly understood but have been interpreted as resembling progressive glomerulonephropathy in rats [67]. Associations with excess dietary protein, underlying chronic viral infections, and renovascular hypertension have been made. Amyloidosis may be concurrent.

Grossly affected kidneys are pale and granular in appearance, with irregular cortical depressions [67]. Histologic changes of the intrarenal vasculature are primarily degenerative, with fibrinoid necrosis occurring in end-stage kidneys [68]. Degeneration of renal tubules is characterized by atrophy or cell regeneration with poorly differentiated epithelium. Glomerular lesions are characterized by segmental to diffuse thickening of basement membranes, with deposition of eosinophilic matrix and at times obliteration of normal structure. The disease may be a major cause of morbidity and mortality, with affected animals experiencing weight loss, polyuria, and polydipsia.

Polycystic disease

Primarily an incidental finding at necropsy, polycystic disease is not uncommon in older hamsters. Single to multiple cysts as large as 2 cm in diameter are found. The liver and epididymis are most commonly affected, but lesions have been reported in the renal pelvis, seminal vesicles, and pancreas. In one colony, it was reported that 76% of hamsters 13 to 27 months old had cystic lesions, and 39% had cysts of various sizes at multiple sites [69].

Neoplasia

Syrian hamsters may develop spontaneous lymphoma or lymphoma associated with hamster papova virus. The kidneys may be involved in multicentric lymphoma. Malaise, anorexia, weight loss, patchy alopecia, and various degrees of palpable abdominal organomegaly have been observed in affected animals.

Gerbil

Gerbils are members of the subfamily Gerbillinae, family Muridae, with 11 to 15 genera and 100 species. The most common pet or laboratory gerbil is the Mongolian gerbil (*Meriones inguiculatus*), a burrowing rodent from the desert regions of China and Mongolia.

Chronic nephropathies as a result of aging are common in gerbils older than 1 year. Gerbils with chronic nephropathy may demonstrate clinical polyuria, polydipsia, and weight loss as the result of decreased appetite. Grossly affected kidneys may be shrunken and show cortical pitting and fibrosis. In a 1995 retrospective study of 141 necropsied gerbils, 16% demonstrated lymphocytic and plasmacytic interstitial nephritis, 18% had chronic tubular nephrosis with eosinophilic proteinaceous or cellular casts in the lumina, and 14% showed chronic glomerulopathy with a variably increased mesangeal matrix, dilated spaces within the Bowman's capsule, and shrunken glomeruli [70]. Other renal lesions included glomerular and interstitial amyloidosis (9%), glomerulosclerosis (6%), pyelonephritis, hydronephrosis, and nephrocalcinosis. This same study revealed renal vascular tumors in aged gerbils; both renal hemangiomas (5% of 141 animals) and hemangiosarcomas (1.5%) were reported. Bacterial nephritis as the result of a *Citrobacter rodentium* septicemia has also been reported in the gerbil [71].

Because of their gnawing behavior, their urine-concentrating ability, and their more efficient nephron, gerbils are prone to accumulations of systemic lead and subsequent toxicity. In an experimental model, the gerbil accumulated four to six times as much renal lead as the rat [72]. Gerbils with chronic toxicity become emaciated; on necropsy, kidneys are grossly small, pale, and pitted. Histologic findings include chronic progressive nephropathy with acid-fast inclusions in proximal collecting tubular epithelium [73]. Development of a microcytic, hypochromic anemia with red blood cell basophilic stippling may aid the diagnosis.

Antemortem diagnosis of renal disease in the gerbil is based on clinical signs (polyuria, polydipsia, weight loss) and serum chemical abnormalities, including elevated serum creatinine concentrations (>1.4 mg/dL) and increased BUN levels (>31.3 mg/dL) [44]. Efforts should be made to rule out a toxic or infectious cause. Treatment involves general renal supportive care, dietary adjustments to reduce protein and phosphorus intake, and specific treatment of any identified underlying cause.

Hedgehogs

Hedgehogs are members of the family Erinaceidae within the order Insectivora. In the pet trade, the African hedgehog (*Atelerix albiventris*) is most commonly seen.

Renal disease is a common finding in the African hedgehog, with one retrospective study showing postmortem histopathologic evidence of renal disease in 50% (7 of 14) of necropsied cases [74]. The histologic classifications in this study included tubulointerstitial nephritis (five of seven), chronic renal infarcts (one of seven), glomerulopathy (one of seven), and tubular nephrosis (one of seven). Gross lesions in this study included tightly adherent renal capsules, irregular and pitted capsular surfaces, granular cut surfaces, multifocal pinpoint pale foci in the renal cortices, and wedge-shaped pale streaks in the renal cortices and medullae [74]. Two of the five hedgehogs with tubulointerstitial nephritis had histologic evidence of systemic inflammatory disease, including septicemia and neoplasia [74]. Potential causes of the presumed primary tubulointerstitial nephritis seen in the other five hedgehogs include an immune-mediated disease, ascending infections, and certain toxins or drugs. Glomerulosclerosis and PKD have also been reported in hedgehogs. Histologic evidence of polycystic kidneys was reported by the Armed Forces Institute of Pathology in one hedgehog in which the renal parenchyma consisted of many dilated tubules lined by a variable squamous-to-cuboidal-to-columnar epithelium and distended by a proteinaceous fluid containing occasional macrophages and degenerate neutrophils. Renal cysts may develop as a result of obstructive lesions (ie, interstitial fibrosis) or exposure to chemicals, or they may be an inherited syndrome. Primary renal neoplasias, including adenocarcinoma and hemangiosarcoma, have been documented on necropsy [75]. Bilateral renal calculi associated with weight loss, azotemia, and hyperphosphatemia have also been reported [76].

Clinical signs of renal disease in the hedgehog are generally nonspecific and include lethargy, anorexia, dehydration, and weight loss. Astute owners may notice polydipsia and polyuria early in renal disease, with absence of water intake occurring in end-stage renal failure. Renomegaly or smaller shrunken kidneys may be seen on radiography/ultrasonography, depending on stage and cause of renal disease. Diagnosis of renal failure is confirmed by urinalysis, CBC, and biochemical analysis. Most cases of degenerative renal disease have been reported in hedgehogs older than 3 years; however, African hedgehogs as young as 7 months have been diagnosed with renal failure [77].

Fluid therapy is an essential aspect of treatment for any animal diagnosed with end-stage renal disease. Many small animals are given long-term fluids by a subcutaneous route to diurese them and control azotemia and uremia. This process may be particularly difficult in the hedgehog because of its short grooved spines that cover the dorsum and its natural defensive behavior of rolling into a tight ball when frightened. This problem was overcome in one case report where a sterile 5-F polyvinylchloride feeding tube (Kendall, Mansfield, Massachusetts) was cut and fenestrated, then tunneled under the skin and sutured in place (Fig. 11) [77]. A luer lock injection plug (Terumo Medical, Elkton, Maryland) was connected to the catheter, through which fluids were easily administered.

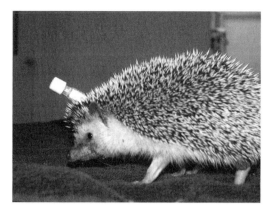

Fig. 11. The owner of this hedgehog was able to diurese at home with subcutaneous fluids. (*From* Powers LV. Subcutaneous implantable catheter for fluid administration in an African pygmy hedgehog. Exotic DVM Veterinary Magazine 2002;4(5):17; with permission.)

Acknowledgments

The author would like to thank Thomas M. Donnelly, BVSc, for his help in reviewing topic outline and providing reference material.

References

[1] Kawasaki TA. Normal parameters and laboratory interpretation of disease states in the domestic ferret. Seminars in Avian and Exotic Pet Medicine 1994;3(1):40–7.

[2] McCrackin Stevenson MA, Gates L, Murray J, et al. Aleutian mink disease parvovirus: implications for companion ferrets. Compendium of Continuing Education 2001;23(6):178–85.

[3] Williams B. Infectious diseases: Aleutian disease. Management of the Ferret for Veterinary Professionals. Proceedings 2000;2:69–70.

[4] Orcutt CJ. Ferret urogenital diseases. Vet Clin North Am Exot Anim Pract 2003;6(1): 113–38.

[5] Nguyen HT, Moreland AF, Shields RP. Urolithiasis in ferrets (*Mustela putorius*). Lab Anim Sci 1979;5:243–5.

[6] Bell RC, Moeller RB. Transitional cell carcinoma of the renal pelvis in a ferret. Lab Anim Sci 1990;40(5):537–8.

[7] Williams BH. Pathology of the domestic ferret (*Mustela putorius furo*). In: 2004 C.L. Davis ACVP Symposium Pathology of Non-Traditional Pets. 2004. p. 103–32.

[8] Richardson JA, Balabuszko RA. Managing ferret toxicosis. Exotic DVM Veterinary Magazine 2000;2(4):23–6.

[9] Cathers TE, Isaza R, Oehme F. Acute ibuprofen toxicosis in a ferret. J Am Vet Med Assoc 2000;216(9):1426–8.

[10] Richardson JA, Balabuszko RA. Ibuprofen ingestion in a ferret. Exotic DVM Veterinary Magazine 2001;3(2):3.

[11] Straube EF, Walden NB. Zinc poisoning in ferrets (*Mustella putoris furo*). Lab Anim 1981; 15(1):45–7.

[12] Straube EF, Schuster NH, Sinclair AJ. Zinc toxicity in the ferret. J Comp Pathol 1980;90(3): 355–61.

[13] Fox JG, Zeman DH, Mortimer JD, et al. Copper toxicosis in sibling ferrets. J Am Vet Med Assoc 1994;205(8):1154–6.

[14] Orcutt CJ, Donnelly TM. Acute ataxia in a ferret following canine distemper vaccination. Lab Anim (NY) 2001;30(9):23–5.

[15] Pollock CG. Urogenital diseases. In: Quesenberry KE, Carpenter JW, editors. Ferrets, rabbits and rodents: clinical medicine and surgery. 2nd edition. Philadelphia: WB Saunders; 2003. p. 41–9.

[16] Dillberger JE. Polycystic kidneys in a ferret. J Am Vet Med Assoc 1985;186(1):74–5.

[17] Fox JA, Parson RC, Bell JA. Diseases of the genitourinary system. In: Fox JG, editor. Biology and diseases of the ferret. Baltimore (MD): Williams & Wilkins; 1998. p. 247–72.

[18] Puerto DA, Walker LM, Saunders HM. Bilateral perinephric pseudocysts and polycystic kidneys in ferrets. Vet Radiol Ultrasound 1988;39(4):309–12.

[19] Marini RP, Taylor NS, Liang AY, et al. Characterization of hemolytic *Escherichia coli* strains in ferrets: recognition of candidate virulence factor CNF1. J Clin Microbiol 2004; 42(12):5904–8.

[20] Rosenbaum MR, Affolter VK, Usborne AL, et al. Cutaneous epitheliotropic lymphoma in a ferret. J Am Vet Med Assoc 1996;209(8):1441–4.

[21] Williams BH, Weiss CA. Ferrets: neoplasia. In: Quesenberry KE, Carpenter JW, editors. Ferrets, rabbits and rodents: clinical medicine and surgery. 2nd edition. Philadelphia: WB Saunders; 2003. p. 91–106.

[22] Li X, Fox JG, Padrid PA. Neoplastic diseases in ferrets: 574 cases (1968–1997). J Am Vet Med Assoc 1998;212(1):1402–6.

[23] Li X, Fox JG. Neoplastic diseases. In: Fox JG, editor. Biology and diseases of the ferret. Baltimore (MD): Williams & Wilkins; 1998. p. 405–47.

[24] Hinton M. Kidney disease in the rabbit: a histological survey. Lab Anim 1981;15:263–5.

[25] Lyngset A. A survey of serum antibodies to *Encephalitozoon cuniculi* in breeding rabbits and their young. Lab Anim Sci 1980;30(3):558–61.

[26] Percy DH, Barthold SW. Rabbit. In: Pathology of laboratory rodents and rabbits. Ames (IA): Blackwell Publishing; 2001. p. 248–306.

[27] Harcourt-Brown FM. *Encephalitozoon cuniculi* in pet rabbits. Vet Rec 2003;152:427–31.

[28] Harcourt-Brown FM. Infectious diseases of domestic rabbits. In: Textbook of rabbit medicine. Oxford (UK): Butterworth Heinemann; 2002. p. 361–85.

[29] Deeb BJ, Carpenter JW. Rabbits: neurologic and musculoskeletal diseases. In: Quesenbery KE, Carpenter JW, editors. Ferrets, rabbits and rodents: clinical medicine and surgery. 2nd edition. Philadelphia: WB Saunders; 2003. p. 203–10.

[30] Harcourt-Brown FM. Urogenital disease. In: Textbook of rabbit medicine. Oxford (UK): Butterworth Heinemann; 2002. p. 335–51.

[31] Redrobe S. Calcium metabolism in rabbits. Seminars in Avian and Exotic Pet Medicine 2002;11(2):94–101.

[32] Pare JA, Paul-Murphy J. Disorders of reproductive and urinary systems. In: Quesenberry KE, Carpenter JW, editors. Ferrets, rabbits and rodents: clinical medicine and surgery. 2nd edition. Philadelphia: WB Saunders; 2003. p. 183–93.

[33] Harris I. The laboratory rabbit facts sheet. ANZCCART News 1994;7(4) [insert].

[34] Zimmerman TE, Giddens WE, DiGiacomo RF, et al. Soft tissue mineralization in rabbits fed a diet containing excess vitamin D. Lab Anim Sci 1990;40:212–5.

[35] Evans KD, Dillehay DL, Huerkamp MJ, et al. Diagnostic exercise: azotemia in a rabbit. Lab Anim Sci 1996;46(4):442–3.

[36] Enriquez JI, Schydlower M, O'Hair K, et al. Effect of vitamin B6 supplementation on gentamicin nephrotoxicity in rabbits. Vet Hum Toxicol 1992;34:32–5.

[37] Wade L. Two uncommonly diagnosed toxins: copper and tremorgenic mycotoxin. In: Proceedings of the AAV Conference. New Orleans (LA): 2004. p. 183–95.

[38] Brammer DW, Doerning BJ, Chrisp CF, et al. Anesthetic and nephrotoxic effects of telazol in New Zealand Whites. Lab Anim Sci 1991;41:432–5.

[39] Gomez L, Gazquez A, Roncero V, et al. Lymphoma in a rabbit: histopathological and immunohistochemical findings. J Small Anim Pract 2002;43(5):224–6.

[40] Lipman NS, Murphy JC, Newcomer CE. Polycythemia in a New Zealand White rabbit with an embryonal nephroma. J Am Vet Med Assoc 1985;187(11):1255–6.

[41] Paul-Murphy J. Urinary tract diseases and disorders. In: Proceedings of the House Rabbit Society Veterinary Conference. Program and abstracts. 1997. p. 53–7.

[42] Xiu-fang H, Ji-shuang C, Xian-giang Y. Effect of tea polyphenols on Masugi nephritis of rabbit. Pak J Biol Sci 2002;5(7):784–8.

[43] Peng X, Griffith JW, Lang CM. Cystitis and cystic calculi in aged guinea pigs. Lab Anim Sci 1987;34:527.

[44] Johnson-Delaney CA. Disease of the urinary system of commonly kept rodents: diagnosis and treatment. Seminars in Avian and Exotic Pet Medicine 1998;7(2):81–8.

[45] Gaschen L, Ketz C, Lang J, et al. Ultrasonographic detection of adrenal gland tumor and ureterolithiasis in a guinea pig. Vet Radiol Ultrasound 1998;39(1):43–6.

[46] Percy DH, Barthold SW. Guinea pig. In: Pathology of laboratory rodents and rabbits. Ames (IA): Blackwell Publishing; 2001. p. 209–47.

[47] Schmidt RE, Reavill DR. The pathology of common diseases in small exotic mammals. In: 2004 C.L. Davis ACVP Symposium Pathology of Non-Traditional Pets. 2004. p. 60–86.

[48] O'Rourke DP. Disease problems of guinea pigs. In: Quesenberry KE, Carpenter JW, editors. Ferrets, rabbits and rodents: clinical medicine and surgery. 2nd edition. Philadelphia: WB Saunders; 2003. p. 245–54.

[49] Kirchner BK, Lake SG, Wrightman SR. Isolation of *Streptobacillus moniloformis* from a guinea pig with granulomatous pneumonia. Lab Anim Sci 1992;42:519–21.

[50] Schoeb TR. Diseases of guinea pigs. PAT 707, Diseases of laboratory animals II, 1989. Available at: http://netvet.wusl.edu/species/guinea/pigs/gpigs.txt. Accessed April 2005.

[51] Boot R, van Knapen F, Kruijt BC, et al. Serological evidence for *Encephalitozoon cuniculi* infection (nosemiasis) in gnotobiotic guinea pigs. Lab Anim (NY) 1988;22:337–42.

[52] Percy DH, Barthold SW. Rats. In: Pathology of laboratory rodents and rabbits. Ames (IA): Blackwell Publishing; 2001. p. 107–67.

[53] Donnelly TM. Diseases of small rodents. In: Quesenberry KE, Carpenter JW, editors. Ferrets, rabbits and rodents: clinical medicine and surgery. 2nd edition. Philadelphia: WB Saunders; 2003. p. 299–315.

[54] Fischer E, Gresh L, Reimann A, et al. Cystic kidney diseases: learning from animal models. Nephrol Dial Transplant 2004;19(11):2700–2.

[55] Casey HW, Irving GW. Bacterial, mycoplasmal, mycotic, and immune-mediated diseases of the urogenital system. In: Foster HL, Small JD, Fox JG, editors. The mouse in biomedical research. Vol. II. Diseases. New York: Academic Press; 1981. p. 43–53.

[56] Percy DH, Barthold SW. Mouse. In: Pathology of laboratory rodents and rabbits. Ames (IA): Blackwell Publishing; 2001. p. 3–106.

[57] Taylor DM, Fraser H, Bruce ME. Altered clinical and histological features of male MM mouse pyelonephritis associated with a change in microbiology. Lab Anim (NY) 1988; 22(1):35–45.

[58] Donnelly T. Sporocysts in the renal epithelium of spiny mice (Acomyscaharinus). Lab Anim (NY) 1999;28(7):23–4.

[59] Schmidt RE. Protozoal diseases of rabbits and rodents. Seminars in Avian and Exotic Pet Medicine 1995;4(3):126–30.

[60] Rosenmann M, Morrison PR. Impairment of metabolic capability in feral house mice by *Klosiella muris* infection. Lab Anim Sci 1975;25:62–4.

[61] Sharma K, McCue P, Dunn SR. Diabetic kidney disease in the db/db mouse. Am J Physiol Renal Physiol 2003;284(6):1138–44.

[62] Yamaguchi M, Manabe N, Uchio-Yamada K, et al. Localization of proliferation and apoptotic cells of ICR-derived glomerulonephritis (ICGN) mice. J Vet Med Sci 2001;63: 781–7.

[63] Dell KN, Li YX, Neilson EG, et al. Localization of the mouse kidney disease (kd) gene to a YAC/BAC contig on Chromosome 10. Mamm Genome 2000;11(11):967–71.
[64] Battles AH. The biology, care, and diseases of the Syrian hamster. Compendium of Continuing Education 1985;7(10):815–23.
[65] Gleiser CA, Van Hoosier GL, Sheldon WG, et al. Amyloidosis and renal paramyloid in a closed hamster colony. Lab Anim Sci 1971;21(2):197–202.
[66] Murphy JC, Fox JG, Niemi SM. Nephrotic syndrome associated with renal amyloidosis in a colony of Syrian hamsters. J Am Vet Med Assoc 1984;185(11):1359–62.
[67] Percy DH, Barthold SW. Hamsters. In: Pathology of laboratory rodents and rabbits. 2nd edition. Ames (IA): Blackwell Publishing; 2001. p. 168–96.
[68] Slauson DO, Hubbs CH, Crain C. Arteriolar sclerosis in the Syrian hamster. Vet Pathol 1978;15(1):1–11.
[69] Gleiser GA, Van Hoosier GL, Sheldon WG. A polycystic disease of hamsters in a closed colony. Lab Anim Care 1970;20(5):923–9.
[70] Bingel SA. Pathologic findings in an aging Mongolian gerbil (Meriones unguiculatus) colony. Lab Anim Sci 1995;45(5):597–600.
[71] de le Puente-Redondo VA, Gutierrez-Marin CB, Perez-Martinez C, et al. Epidemic infection caused by Citrobacter rodentium in a gerbil colony. Vet Rec 1999;145(14):400–3.
[72] Vincent AL, Rodrick GE, Sodeman WA. The pathology of the Mongolian gerbil (Meriones unguiculatus) colony. Lab Anim Sci 1979;29(5):645–51.
[73] Percy DH, Barthold SW. Gerbils. In: Pathology of laboratory rodents and rabbits. 2nd edition. Ames (IA): Blackwell Publishing; 2001. p. 197–208.
[74] Raymond JT, White MR. Necropsy and histopathologic findings in 14 African hedgehogs (Atelerix albiventris): a retrospective study. J Zoo Wildl Med 1999;30(2):273–7.
[75] Done LB. What you don't know about hedgehog diseases. In: North American Veterinary Conference Proceedings. 1999. p. 824–5.
[76] Johnson DH. Hedgehog with suspected bilateral renal calculi. Exotic DVM Veterinary Magazine 2001;3(1):6.
[77] Powers LV. Subcutaneous implantable catheter for fluid administration in an African pygmy hedgehog. Exotic DVM Veterinary Magazine 2002;4(5):16–7.

VETERINARY
CLINICS
Exotic Animal Practice

ELSEVIER
SAUNDERS

Vet Clin Exot Anim 9 (2006) 69–96

Exotic Mammal Renal Disease: Diagnosis and Treatment

Peter G. Fisher, DVM

*Pet Care Veterinary Hospital, 5201-A Virginia Beach Boulevard,
Virginia Beach, VA 23462, USA*

The kidneys of most mammals, including the ferret, are multipapillate. By contrast, the kidneys of rodents and rabbits are uniquely unipapillate, with one papilla and one calyx forming the renal pelvis that narrows to enter the ureter directly. In ferrets, rabbits, and rodents, the kidney is the typical bean-shaped organ lying in sublumbar retroperitoneal space, with the cranial pole of the right kidney situated at the level of T14 and the cranial pole of the left kidney approximately at the level of L1. Rabbit kidneys generally sit lower in the abdomen than those of ferrets, in which the dorsal surface of the kidneys is in direct contact with the sublumbar muscles in the retroperitoneal space [1]. The urinary bladder and ureters are as in the dog and cat.

At the microscopic level, the nephron length may vary from species to species and even within a given kidney, but they are all composed of the same segments [2]. The nephron begins with the renal corpuscle or glomerulus, which leads into the proximal convoluted tubule followed by the distal convoluted tubule. The distal tubule leads into the tubule that connects the nephron to the cortical collecting duct, which descends straight to the renal medulla, coalesces there with other collecting ducts, and finally terminates at the papillary tip. The urine literally drips from the collecting ducts, where it is collected by the renal calyces; these coalesce to form the renal pelvis, which narrows to form the ureter [2].

The natural environment of the species in question has a strong influence on both the internal organization and consequent size of the kidney. As a general rule, desert-dwelling species, such as hamsters and gerbils, have large kidneys with powerful urine-concentrating ability. A larger renal medulla in these species allows the kidney to respond to water deprivation by extracting more water from the fluid within the tubules and returning this fluid to the plasma [2]. The ratio of medulla to cortex in the gerbil is

E-mail address: peter.g.fisher@verizon.net

doi:10.1016/j.cvex.2005.10.002
vetexotic.theclinics.com

approximately twice that of the laboratory rat [3]. This factor explains the high specific gravity of urine in these species and their ability to obtain most, if not all, of their water requirements from metabolic processes and any available fruit or vegetable matter [4]. The same is true for rabbits, in that those from desert zones have large kidneys as compared with those from alpine zones [5].

Terminology

Many different and sometimes confusing terms are used to describe renal function and its deterioration [6].

- *Azotemia* refers to an increased concentration of urea nitrogen, creatinine, and other nonproteinaceous nitrogenous waste products in the blood. *Renal azotemia* denotes azotemia caused by renal parenchymal changes [6].
- *Uremia* is the presence of all urine constituents in the blood. Usually a toxic condition, it may occur secondary to renal failure or postrenal disorders, including urethral blockage.
- *Renal reserve* may be viewed as the percentage of "extra" nephrons, those not necessary to maintain normal renal function [6]. Although this figure probably varies from animal to animal, it is greater than 50% in most mammals.
- *Renal insufficiency* begins when the renal reserve is lost. Animals with renal insufficiency outwardly appear normal but have a reduced capacity to compensate for stresses, such as infection or dehydration, and have lost urine-concentrating ability [6].
- *Renal failure* is a state of decreased renal function that enables persistent abnormalities (azotemia and inability to concentrate urine) to exist; it refers to a level of organ function rather than a specific disease entity [6].

Most of the renal diseases discussed in these articles can manifest as various stages of compromise in renal reserve, as renal insufficiency, or as renal failure. The timing and potential for progression of the disease process depend on variables that include the specific disease in question, environmental factors, and the individual animal. Clinical techniques used to assess renal health include blood serum and urine analysis, survey radiography, ultrasonography, and other imaging modalities.

Specimen collection

Cystocentesis by a ventral midline approach is the preferred method of urine collection. Because of the thin bladder wall of exotic mammals, patient sedation and use of a 23-gauge, 1-in needle in rabbits and ferrets and a 25-gauge needle in smaller species is preferred to avoid inadvertent bladder wall laceration and subsequent urine leakage. Three to six mL of urine provide enough volume for a thorough urinalysis. Manual expression and free-catch samples may be used but are less than ideal owing to vaginal, preputial, and environmental contamination. Urethral catheterization is difficult in the ferret because of anatomy. (See the section on urolithiasis and obstructive disease.) Catheterization of the urethra is possible in male and female rabbits using a 3.5 to 9 F catheter and sedation with midazolam (1 mg/kg intramuscularly) or gas inhalant anesthesia. The male rabbit is restrained in a sitting position to extrude the penis, and the catheter is passed approximately 1 in into the urethra to obtain a sample (Fig. 1) [7]. The urethral os of the female rabbit is located on the floor of the vagina and is best accessed with the rabbit in sternal recumbency [7].

For blood collection, emphasis is placed on using the safest and least traumatic method. The author prefers the vena cava or other large veins accessed at the sternal notch in ferrets, guinea pigs, and hedgehogs, and the lateral saphenous vein in rabbits and rats (Fig. 2). A 25-gauge needle placed in the lateral saphenous vein followed by capillary tube collection works well in smaller species, such as hamsters, gerbils, and mice. Depending on species and animal temperament, anesthesia is often preferred to avoid accidental trauma. Newer chemistry analyzers or outside laboratories specializing in exotic species allow for serum chemistry and complete blood count results on minimal (100-μL) volumes of blood. It is estimated that 10% of blood volume (55–70 mL/kg body weight) may be safely taken for blood sampling every 3 to 4 weeks [8].

Clinical pathology

Hematology, clinical chemistry, and urinalysis values may vary significantly with strain or breed of animal, nutritional status, sex, sampling site

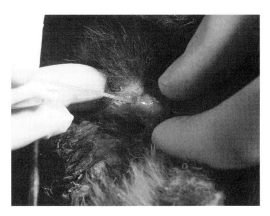

Fig. 1. This male rabbit has been anesthetized using isoflurane and the penis extended so as successfully to pass a 3.5 F tomcat catheter for urine collection.

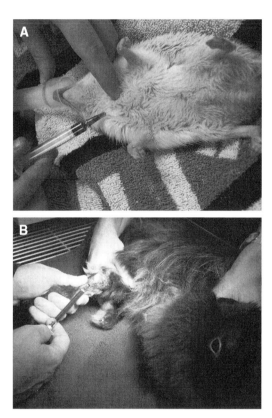

Fig. 2. For blood collection the author prefers the vena cava or other large veins accessed at the sternal notch in ferrets, guinea pigs, and hedgehogs. This hedgehog (*A*) has been anesthetized to allow access and to avoid potential accidental trauma, and successful blood draw has been achieved using a 3-mL syringe with a 22-gauge 0.75-in needle. The laternal saphenous vein is being used in the rabbit on the left (*B*) to collect blood using a 1-mL tuberculin syringe with a 25-gauge 0.625-in needle.

or frequency, time of day, stressors, age, health status, drug exposure, and environment [8]. Therefore, normal values are broad, and these variabilities should be kept in mind when interpreting individual animal values (Table 1).

Evaluation of renal function in exotic mammals is similar to that in dogs and cats, with some exceptions that will be detailed in this section. Glomerular function is evaluated by determination of blood urea nitrogen (BUN) and serum creatinine concentrations, which are both freely filtered through the glomerular basement membrane [9]. Filtered urea, an end-product of protein catabolism, is reabsorbed through the renal tubules, whereas creatinine, an end-product of muscle metabolism, is released in the circulation at a constant rate and does not undergo tubular resorption. The BUN concentration is inversely proportional to the glomerular filtration rate, but BUN is not produced and excreted at a constant rate [1]. BUN serum levels are influenced

Table 1
Normal serum chemistry values frequently associated with renal disease

	Blood urea nitrogen (mg/dL)	Creatinine (mg/dL)	Phosphorus (mg/dL)	Calcium (mg/dL)
Ferret	10–45	0.4–0.9	4.0–9.1	8.0–11.8
Rabbit	13–29	0.5–2.5	0.5–2.5	5.6–12.5
Guinea pig	9.0–31.5	0.6–2.2	3.0–7.6	8.2–12.0
Hedgehog	13–54	0.4–0.8	2.4–12.0	5.2–11.3
Mouse	27.5–34.7	0.74–1.01	10.4–13.8	10.7–12.4
Rat	15–21	0.2–0.8	5.3–8.3	5.3–13.0
Hamster	12–25	0.91–0.99	3.4–8.2	5–12
Gerbil	17–27	0.6–1.4	3.7–6.2	3.7–6.1

Data from Refs. [4,8,14]; Ivey E, Carpenter JW. African hedgehogs. In: Quesenberry KE, Carpenter JW, editors. Ferrets, rabbits and rodents: clinical medicine and surgery. 2nd edition. Philadelphia: WB Saunders; 2004. p. 339–53; Ness RD. Clinical pathology and sample collection of exotic small mammals. Vet Clin North Am Exot Anim pract 1999;2:591–620.

by protein levels in the diet, liver function, intestinal bleeding and subsequent nitrogen absorption, and the state of hydration. Because the BUN may be influenced by nonrenal factors, creatinine generally serves as a better indicator of renal function. Unfortunately, increases in serum concentrations of both substances do not occur until an estimated 75% of renal function has been lost, making early diagnosis of many renal diseases difficult.

When evaluating azotemia in exotic mammals, one should establish whether it is prerenal, primary renal, or postrenal in origin. A physical examination that assesses hydration, renal discomfort, size and shape of kidneys and bladder, abdominal masses, and urinary obstruction will help form the basis for further diagnostics [10]. Prerenal azotemia occurs when there is decreased renal perfusion (dehydration, shock, or cardiac disease) or as a result of a high-protein diet or intestinal hemorrhage [1]. Prerenal azotemia is common in rabbits and is found in association with stress, fright, water deprivation, severe dehydration, heat stroke, and toxic insults [11]. The rabbit has a limited capacity to concentrate urea; therefore, dehydration may readily result in elevated (prerenal) values of BUN and creatinine that might be associated with renal disease in other species. This finding was substantiated in one retrospective study of 190 rabbits seen in Japan from 1998 to 2001 with BUN values greater than 27 mg/dL, where the majority of cases involved gastrointestinal disorder (54 cases) and overgrowth of molar teeth, diseases capable of causing stress and dehydration [12]. In most cases of prerenal azotemia, elevations in BUN are less than 100 mg/dL and are accompanied by an increase in urine specific gravity greater than 1.03.

Primary or renal azotemia occurs with renal parenchymal disease and glomerular damage and is accompanied by variable increases in BUN and creatinine levels and isosthenuric urine. Postrenal azotemia occurs with urinary tract obstruction, most commonly due to calculi. The urine specific gravity may vary in cases of postrenal azotemia.

Ferrets are unique in that their creatinine levels (0.2–0.6 mg/dL) are considerably lower than in other mammals and have a narrower range (0.2–0.9 mg/dL). As a result, serum creatinine levels that may be considered high in ferrets can still be within the normal range for other species [13]. Mechanisms of creatinine excretion other than free glomerular filtration, such as renal tubular secretion or greater enteric degradation, may play a larger role in this species [9]. Consequently, elevations in the concentration of BUN associated with renal failure are not always accompanied by increases in the concentration of serum creatinine above the normal range. Any increase in serum creatinine above normal should be considered significant in the ferret. BUN measurements of greater than 100 mg/dL with a concurrent creatinine of 2.0 mg/dL would be consistent with significant renal disease in the ferret. Creatinine and inulin clearance can be used to measure glomerular filtration rate and detect early renal insufficiency in ferrets, although this is impractical in private practice because it requires either metabolic cages or placement of an indwelling catheter [9]. Creatinine and inulin clearance values in the ferret have been reported as 3.32 mL/min/kg and 3.02 mL/min/kg, respectively [9].

Circulating levels of phosphorus are largely controlled by the kidneys, and consistent elevations in phosphorus in the face of isosthenuria and azotemia are not uncommon in animals with renal failure. Vitamin D and parathyroid hormone influence intestinal absorption of phosphorus; parathyroid hormone stimulates renal excretion of phosphorus and conservation of calcium. The hyperphosphatemia that occurs in chronic renal failure is closely related to dietary protein intake inasmuch as protein-rich diets are also high in phosphorus. Therefore, one can assume that carnivores such as the ferret are likely to develop the hyperphosphatemia and renal secondary hyperparathyroidism seen in canine and feline chronic renal failure. Hyperphosphatemia is also seen in rabbits with kidney disease as a result of impaired renal phosphorus excretion [14].

Other clinicopathologic abnormalities associated with renal failure include red blood cell (RBC) suppression, acidosis, hyperkalemia, and hypo- or hypercalcemia. Anemia of chronic renal failure is a common entity and results from reduced erythropoietin production by damaged kidneys, uremic inhibition of RBC production, and increased RBC hemolysis [15]. In rabbits with chronic renal failure, hypercalcemia may occur as a result of impaired renal calcium excretion [14]. It has also been noted secondary to experimentally induced chronic renal failure [16].

The urinalysis offers practitioners an excellent tool for assessing urinary tract health and should be performed in any exotic mammals with suspected renal disease (Table 2). The specific gravity may help differentiate prerenal from renal azotemia, as reviewed previously. Urine protein may be elevated with urinary tract inflammation, hemorrhage, or infection or may indicate renal damage. Protein levels in the urine must be interpreted along with the urine specific gravity and sediment analysis [1]. Glomerulonephritis

Table 2
Normal urinalysis results from exotic mammals

	Specific gravity	Protein (mg/dL)	pH	Urine volume (mL/24 h)
Ferret	N/A	0–33	6.5–7.5	26–140
Rabbit	1.003–1.036	Trace	8.2–8.8	130/kg
Guinea pig	N/A	N/A	9.0	N/A
Mouse	1.034–1.058	N/A	7.3–8.5	0.5–2.5
Rat	1.022–1.050	<30	7.0–7.4	13–23
Hamster	1.050–1.060	N/A	Basic	5.1–8.4
Gerbil	N/A	N/A	N/A	Few drops–4 mL

Abbreviation: N/A, not available.
Data from Refs. [4,7,13]; McClure DE. Clinical pathology and sample collection in the laboratory rodent. Vet Clin North Am Exot Anim Pract 1999;2:565–90.

and amyloidosis are the most common causes of renally associated proteinuria. Healthy adult rabbits and ferrets may have trace-to-small amounts of proteinuria. Healthy adult mice have a normal proteinuria, with higher levels seen in sexually mature mice [17]. Proteinuria is normal in rats owing to tubular production of alpha globulins, with urine protein levels as great as 30 mg/dL [18]. Proteinuria is normal in adult hamsters, but excessive levels of urine protein are commonly associated with renal amyloidosis. Small amounts of protein can normally be found in a gerbil's scant and concentrated urine.

Hematuria may result from upper or lower urinary tract disease or be of uterine origin in intact females. Hematuria of renal origin is seen in pyelonephritis, neoplasia, renoliths, and renal infarcts.

Urine sediment analysis can offer information on urinary tract hemorrhage, inflammation, and bacteria. Bacteriuria may be an indication of upper or lower urinary tract infection but is more commonly associated with lower urinary tract disease. Keep in mind that bacteriuria may also be associated with prostatic or uterine infections. Bacterial culture with antimicrobial sensitivity testing is warranted in any case of bacteriuria. Casts are cylindric molds of the renal tubules; they are composed of aggregates of proteins and cells and may indicate a pathologic change in the kidneys [1]. Granular casts are composed of degenerative cells, plasma proteins, and other substances (eg, lipids); in large numbers they are indicative of active renal tubular cell injury. Increased numbers of leucocytes in the urine sediment, especially neutrophils, indicate nonspecific urinary tract inflammation, whereas white blood cell casts are suggestive of pyelonephritis. Renal epithelial cell casts, which suggest tubular sloughing, may occur with acute tubular necrosis or pyelonephritis [1].

Imaging

Plain abdominal radiography can assess for increases or decreases in kidney size, radiopaque calculi within the urinary tract, abdominal masses associated with the urinary tract, and bladder distention (Fig. 3). The kidneys and urinary tract of the smallest exotic mammals (rodents) are hard to discern on plain radiographs, making contrast urography a useful tool in assessing renal anomalies and other abnormalities. One report describes the use of the lateral saphenous vein for administration of contrast material to perform intravenous pyelograms in rats [19]. Contrast cystography and urethrography can provide more specific information regarding the bladder and urethra. Intravenous pyelograms or excretory urography is used to evaluate the size, shape, position, and internal structure of the kidneys, ureter, and urinary bladder and is especially helpful in assessing the upper urinary tract (kidneys and ureters) for calculi, masses, or obstructive lesions [20]. Iohexol (240 mg iodine/mL), at a dose of 720 mg iodine/kg injected into a cephalic catheter, is one iodinated contrast material used in ferrets for excretory urography [20].

Renal ultrasonography plays a role in discerning tissue architecture, allowing for differentiation between focal and diffuse disease and between

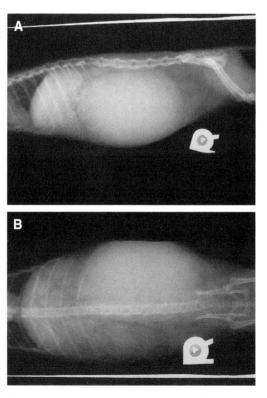

Fig. 3. This female ferret was presented for an abdominal swelling noticed by the owner. Radiographs revealed a larger radiodense mass in the mid-right abdomen. (*A*) Lateral abdominal. (*B*) Ventro-dorsal abdominal. BUN and creatinine were normal. Exploratory surgery revealed a unilateral hydronephrotic kidney, presumably the result of inadvertent urethral ligation at the time of ovariohysterectomy.

echodense and echolucent lesions (Fig. 4). Ultrasonography can help with the diagnosis of pyelonephritis, hydronephrosis, and hydroureter, as well as that of renal cysts and abscesses.

The author refers readers to other sources for details on performing urinary tract contrast studies, catheterization techniques, and interpretation of sonograms.

General treatment for chronic renal failure

Many of the diseases discussed in Fisher's article on etiology and clinical presentation of exotic mammal renal disease in this issue can progress to renal failure. Depending on the specific progression of renal failure and uremia, the patient may present in various states of lethargy, decreased appetite or total anorexia, increased or decreased water intake, dehydration, and general malaise. Concurrent gastrointestinal upset (stasis in herbivores) is not uncommon.

Once a diagnosis is made, general treatment guidelines for animals with chronic renal failure include those listed in Box 1.

The author refers readers to an exotic pharmacology formulary [21] for more specific information on drug dosing and frequency.

Urolithiasis and obstructive disease

Treatment of urolithiasis varies with stone location and severity of disease. Urethral obstruction and subsequent postrenal failure may usually be diagnosed based on clinical signs, physical examination findings, and

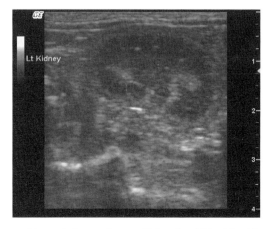

Fig. 4. This ultrasound image is from a 2-year-old female rabbit with a history of weight loss, polyuria/polydipsia, and slight ataxia. The rabbit had a positive *E cuniculi* titer. (Courtesy of Alessandro Melillo, DVM.)

Box 1. General treatment guidelines for animals with chronic renal failure

- Discontinue any potentially nephrotoxic drugs.
- Identify and treat any prerenal or postrenal abnormalities.
- Identify any treatable conditions, such as urolithiasis or pyelonephritis.
- Improve or modify the diet as appropriate for the species.
- If animal is hyperphosphatemic, initiate enteric phosphate binders.
- Treat gastroenteritis, if present, with metoclopromide or H_2 blockers.
- Treat anemia with vitamin/iron supplementation or human recombinant erythropoietin.
- Provide caloric requirements.
- Initiate intravenous fluid therapy to reduce azotemia in those species in which intravenous catheters may be placed (Fig. 5). Follow up with maintenance subcutaneous fluid therapy (Fig. 6) (owners may be taught to do this at home). Volumes given vary with patient size: 50 to 60 mL per injection site in rabbits and ferrets, 30 to 35 mL in guinea pigs, 20 to 25 mL in hedgehogs, 10 to 15 mL in rats, 3 to 5 mL in mice, gerbils, and hamsters. Normal daily water intake in ferrets, rabbits, and guinea pigs is estimated to be 100 mL/kg.
- In any patient with renal failure, quality of life issues and euthanasia should be discussed with the owner.
- Consider use of omega-3 fatty acid supplements.

Note: Renal-friendly dietary changes are difficult in many exotic mammals as a result of specific dietary requirements or olfactory imprinting, which determines dietary preference at an early age.

---

imaging by radiologic or ultrasound examination of the caudal abdomen (Fig. 7). Clinical signs of urethral obstruction are similar to those in other mammalian species and include stranguria, dysuria, pollakiuria, and hematuria, with eventual anorexia, lethargy, and abdominal pain. If not corrected, urethral obstruction can lead to severe metabolic disorder, coma, and death (Fig. 8) [10]. Affected animals are usually dehydrated, listless, and hunched owing to abdominal pain. Abdominal palpation reveals an enlarged turgid bladder. Acute renal failure secondary to urethral obstruction may be diagnosed by abnormalities in the biochemical profile, including elevated BUN and creatinine levels, hyperphosphatemia, and hyperkalemia. Most cases of urethral obstruction also demonstrate a hemorrhagic cystitis, usually accompanied by a urinary bacterial infection. Urine bacterial culture

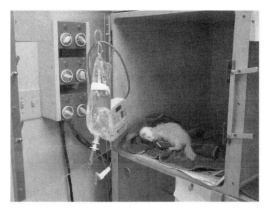

Fig. 5. Patients who have uremia should be hospitalized and intravenous fluid therapy and correction of metabolic imbalances instituted. This ferret was hypothermic and has been set up in an incubated cage, with a cephalic catheter placed. An infusion pump is essential to administer the low volumes of intravenous fluids required by exotic mammals. (*From* Fisher PG. Equipping the exotic mammal practice. Vet Clin North Am Exot Anim Pract 2005;8(3):413; with permission.)

and antimicrobial sensitivity testing are warranted in all cases of obstructive uropathy.

When approaching urethral obstruction in ferrets, one must assess for prostatomegaly and periprostatic cysts in male ferrets and for periurethral cysts in either sex and rule out underlying neoplasia. If primary adrenal disease and resultant secondary obstructive gross pyuria, prostatomegaly, or periprostatic cysts are suspected, then one should consider ultrasonography to assess adrenal gland size or submit an adrenal hormone panel to the University of Tennessee. Pathognomonic signs of adrenal disease, such as various degrees of alopecia, pruritus, or behavioral changes (aggression or

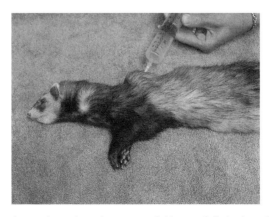

Fig. 6. Owners can be taught to give subcutaneous fluids on a daily basis to diurese ferrets that have azotemia resulting from chronic renal failure.

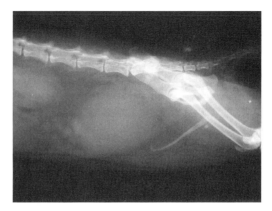

Fig. 7. A urethral calculus causing obstruction can be seen just proximal to the os penis in this lateral radiograph of a male ferret. This ferret showed clinial signs of dysuria and abdominal pain and was suffering from postrenal azotemia.

increased sexual activity), may help confirm a suspicion. Medical or surgical therapy for adrenal disease prevents recurrence of future secondary obstructive disease. The author refers readers to other sources for detailed information on treatment of ferret adrenal disease and secondary complications.

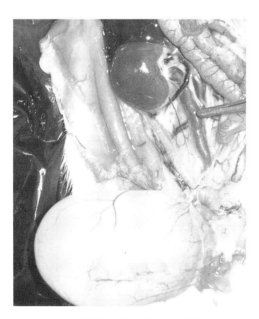

Fig. 8. This Long-Evans rat had urolithiasis that obstructed the urethra, preventing urination. On necropsy it was found that the obstruction resulted in bladder distention and subsequent hydroureter (*arrow*) with distention of the renal pelvis. (*From* Coria-Avila GA, Barbosa-Vargas E, Pfaus JG. Sudden bladder distention in a female rat. Lab Animal 2005;34(6):22; with permission.)

Struvite urolithiasis is another cause of urethral blockage in ferrets and has been associated with feeding a commercial pelleted canine diet [22]. Converting ferrets to a high-quality animal protein–based diet will acidify the urine and aid in prevention of magnesium ammonium phosphate calculi, the most commonly reported urinary tract calculi in ferrets.

Treatment for acute renal failure secondary to urethral obstruction involves relief of the obstruction, followed by fluid diuresis, analgesia, and correction of electrolyte imbalances, secondary gastrointestinal disturbances, and bacterial cystitis. The options available for relieving the obstruction include cystocentesis, urethral catheterization, urethrotomy, and placement of a cystostomy catheter. Urethral catheterization of the male ferret is complicated by the J-shaped os penis, the narrow diameter of the penile urethra, and the acute bend of the urethra at the pelvic canal [23]. The author uses a 3 F, 11-cm open-ended silicone urinary catheter (Slippery Sam, Surgivet, Inc., Waukesha, WI) to catheterize and flush the urethra (Fig. 9A). Initial catheterization may be aided by retrograde flushing through a blunt needle placed in the urethral orifice opening to dilate the urethra and allow for placement of a closed-ended urinary catheter (Fig. 9B) [24].

Urethral calculus obstruction may be relieved by anesthetizing the patient and using a urethral catheter to flush the calculus into the bladder, followed by removal by cystotomy. If one is unsuccessful at dislodging the calculus, perineal urethrostomy may be performed (Fig. 10).

A tube cystostomy has also been advocated as a means of providing urine outflow and relieving the immediate cause of acute renal failure. Its use has been described in four ferrets with a history of preoperative urinary obstruction, nonexpressable bladders, and prostatomegaly, prostatic cysts, or periurethral swelling identified at adrenalectomy surgery [25]. During exploratory celiotomy, a 5 or 8 F Foley catheter was passed through a ventral abdominal paramedian incision and then into the bladder lumen, where it was secured with a purse-string suture.

The long-term prognosis for exotic mammals with bilateral renal calculi is guarded. Supportive treatment includes analgesia, appetite stimulants, antibiotics as indicated, and demonstration to owners of how to administer daily or every-other-day subcutaneous fluids. Indications for surgical removal of nephroliths include obstruction of the renal pelvis and urine outflow, chronic recurrent urinary tract infection associated with nephrolithiasis, substantial increase in size of nephroliths in symptomatic patients, and progressive deterioration of renal function [26]. Surgical procedures vary with size and location of the nephrolith and include nephrotomy (Fig. 11), pyelolithotomy, and nephrectomy. The surgeon needs to be aware that incising renal parenchyma results in destruction of some nephrons, both as a direct result of the incision and indirectly from severing of blood vessels and increased pressure imposed by the hemorrhage and transudation associated with surgery [27]. Bilateral nephrotomy should be avoided, because studies in dogs have shown an overall postnephrotomy

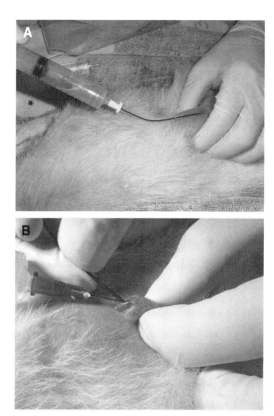

Fig. 9. This ferret suffered from postrenal azotemia secondary to urethral compression as a result of prostatic hyperplasia secondary to adrenal disease. (*A*) A 3 F, 11-cm open-ended silicone urinary catheter (Slippery Sam, Surgivet, Inc., Waukesha, WI) is used to catheterize and flush the urethra. (*From* Fisher PG. Equipping the exotic mammal practice. Vet Clin North Am Exot Anim Pract 2005;8(3):415; with permission.) (*B*) Initial catheterization may be aided by the use of retrograde flushing through a blunt needle placed in the urethral orifice opening to dilate the urethra and allow for placement of the closed-ended urinary catheter.

complication rate of 33.8% and a 20% to 40% decline in glomerular filtration rate as compared with presurgical values [27]. All animals undergoing nephrotomy should have urine production measured during and after surgery to assure normal function in the contralateral kidney. A ureterotomy may be performed for retrieval of unilateral ureteroliths, but this is a microsurgical procedure best performed with the aid of an operating microscope and 6-0 or 7-0 absorbable suture. Alternatively, a nephrectomy may be performed in small exotic mammals with unilateral ureteral or renal pelvic calculi causing obstruction and hydronephrosis.

Preventive measures to control recurrence of rabbit urolithiasis include dietary modifications, weight loss, use of distilled drinking water, and oral potassium citrate to reduce urinary calcium concentrations. Feeding lower-calcium grass hays, timothy-based pellets, and leafy green

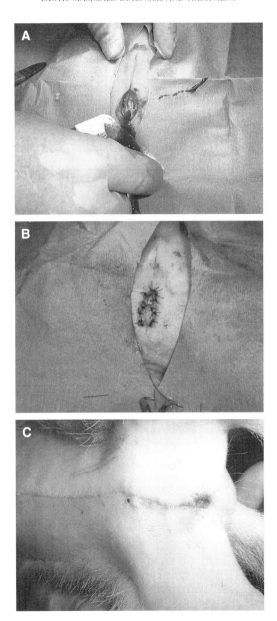

Fig. 10. A perineal urethrostomy has been performed on this ferret to relieve a lower urinary tract obstruction caused by several urethral calculi that the author was unable to flush retrograde into the bladder for removal. The obstruction resulted in postrenal azotemia (*A*,*B*). Fluid diuresis and supportive care postoperatively resulted in uneventful healing (*C*).

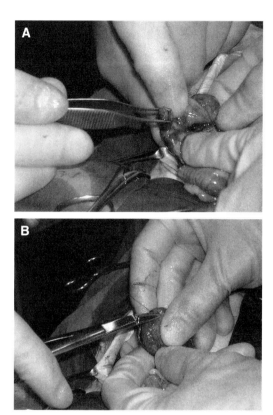

Fig. 11. (A,B) A nephrotomy was performed in this rabbit for the successful removal of unilateral renal pelvis calculi. This rabbit presented for abdominal pain and perineal dermal scalding secondary to urinary incontinence. Renal function was normal preoperatively. (Courtesy of William Lewis, BVSc, MRCVS.)

vegetables will help reduce calcium intake and consequently help control hypercalciuria.

Distal ureteral calculi are not uncommon in the guinea pig; therefore, multiple views are recommended when performing plain radiography to delineate anatomic location of calculi. Ultrasonography has been used to diagnose a calcium carbonate ureterolith as a cause of ureteral obstruction and subsequent hydronephrosis in the guinea pig [28]. Medical and surgical treatment of urolithiasis has been disappointing in the guinea pig because the exact mechanism of calculi formation is unknown, making dissolution impossible, prevention difficult, and recurrence after surgical removal common. Suggested recommendations for medical treatment include antibiotics to control infection, pain management, and dietary modifications [29]. Foods containing high levels of oxalates (eg, spinach, parsley, celery, strawberries) should be avoided. Potassium citrate has been advocated in stone prevention because of its capacity to bind calcium, reduce ion activity, and inhibit crystal formation. The enteric oxalate-using bacterium *Oxalobacter formigenes* may play a role in the prevention of hyperoxaluria in some rodent species [29].

Space-occupying renal lesions

Diagnosis of space-occupying renal lesions, such as hydronephrosis, renal cysts and abscesses, pyelonephritis, and neoplasia, benefits from the use of ultrasonography to assess renal architecture. Physical examination findings, clinical pathology, radiographic contrast studies, and fine needle aspirate cytology are additional tools used to make a definitive diagnosis in these cases.

Hydronephrosis

Diagnosis of hydronephrosis is made by abdominal palpation of an enlarged kidney or abdominal mass and confirmed radiographically as a uniformly radiopaque unilateral, midabdominal mass. Ultrasonography or intravenous pyelography will help confirm the diagnosis (Fig. 12). Imaging techniques also help with diagnosis of hydroureter and underlying causes of ureter blockage. Urine, complete blood count, and biochemical analysis help determine contralateral kidney function and rule out secondary urinary tract bacterial infection. Analysis of fluid removed from the hydronephrotic kidney by means of a fine needle aspirate will reveal a transudate unless secondary bacterial infection is present [30].

Unilateral nephrectomy carries a good prognosis if the remaining kidney function is normal. If the condition is secondary to ureteral calculi, stone analysis should be performed and measures taken to prevent recurrence.

Renal cysts

Most renal cysts are found incidentally on necropsy or ultrasonography and do not cause clinical disease. Ferrets with polycystic kidney disease (PKD) that progress to renal failure may be presented for anorexia, weight loss, gastrointestinal dysfunction, and significant lethargy. Physical examination and abdominal palpation in these cases may reveal a midabdominal mass or masses. Follow-up radiographs usually demonstrate two soft tissue radiopacities consistent with grossly enlarged kidneys. Renal failure and its associated clinical pathology may be confirmed with a complete blood count, biochemical analysis, and urinalysis. Pyelography with intravenous contrast media or nuclear scintigraphy may be useful to evaluate renal function in some clinically affected ferrets [30]. Abdominal ultrasonography may be used to confirm PKD, determine the extent of disease, and rule out perinephric pseudocysts.

No specific treatment for renal cysts exists. If cysts are found on ultrasound examination, ferrets should be assessed for renal function and then

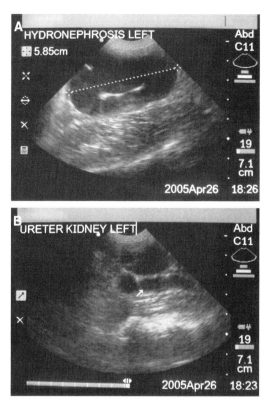

Fig. 12. These ultrasound images are from a rabbit that presented with a palpable abdominal mass. Ultrasonography revealed a unilateral left-sided hydronephrosis (*A*) and hydroureter (*B*). On surgical exploration, the left ureter was found to be constricted by a band of fibrosis of unknown origin. (Courtesy of William Lewis, BVSc, MRCVS.)

monitored periodically for development of more cysts by means of abdominal palpation, ultrasonography, biochemical analysis, and urinalysis. In humans, renal cysts have been associated with pain and hematuria [30]. If pain associated with a large renal cyst is suspected, a unilateral nephrectomy may be performed if contralateral kidney function is determined to be adequate (Fig. 13). Renal failure associated with polycystic kidney disease generally carries a poor prognosis. Supportive and general renal failure treatment may be attempted.

Pyelonephritis

Differentiating cystitis and lower urinary tract disease from pyelonephritis can be difficult. Box 2 summarizes clinical findings associated with pyelonephritis. Animals with cystitis may show various degrees of dysuria, stranguria, and pollakiuria but otherwise are clinically normal. Animals with pyelonephritis usually show an acute onset of fever, lethargy, anorexia,

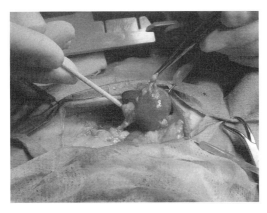

Fig. 13. This large renal cyst was causing pain in this 5-year-old female ferret. Clinical pathology indicated normal renal function, and a unilateral nephrectomy was performed, resolving the abdominal pain.

and pain on palpation of kidneys. Clinical pathology can also help differentiate the two syndromes, and blood should be submitted for a complete blood count and serum biochemical analysis; urine should be collected sterilely by cystocentesis or ultrasound-guided pyelocentesis and submitted for urinalysis and bacterial culture with antimicrobial sensitivity testing. Pyelonephritis may result in a leukocytosis characterized by a left shift or mature neutrophilia. Depending on severity and degree of renal involvement, BUN and creatinine may or may not be elevated. Cases of chronic untreated pyelonephritis resulting in end-stage chronic renal failure will demonstrate isosthenuria, azotemia, and hyperphosphatemia. Examination of urine sediment may show increased numbers of white blood cells (especially neutrophils), bacteria, red blood cells, and renal tubular or white blood cell casts. Ultrasound or an intravenous pyelogram may help confirm pyelonephritis.

Box 2. Clinical and pathologic findings associated with pyelonephritis in exotic small mammals

- Leukocytosis, fever
- Renal pain on abdominal palpation
- Renal failure: azotemia, isosthenuria
- Cellular casts in urine sediment
- Bacteriuria with positive urine culture
- Positive bacterial culture of ultrasound-guided fluid aspirate from renal pelvis (pyelocentesis)
- Excretory urogram or ultrasonography abnormalities, including renal pelvis dilatation, dilated ureters, or asymmetric filling of renal diverticula

On necropsy, diagnosis is ideally based on tissue culture results, accompanied by the histologic demonstration of bacteria within the lesions. Smears from fresh lesions stained for bacteria will often permit a rapid, presumptive diagnosis.

Treatment for pyelonephritis includes fluid therapy and diuresis, nutritional support, and antibiotics based on sensitivity results. Parenteral antibiotics are recommended during initial treatment, followed by 4 to 6 weeks of oral antibiotic therapy. Post-treatment culture of a sterilely collected urine specimen is recommended to ensure that the bacterial infection has been eliminated, and biochemical parameters should be monitored for resolution of any pre-existing azotemia. Treatment of underlying urolithiasis or causative adrenal disease is essential in prevention of recurrence.

Neoplasia

Clinical signs of urinary tract neoplasia include hematuria, dysuria, incontinence, anorexia, lethargy, and weight loss. Abdominal palpation, radiography, urinalysis, ultrasonography, and ultrasound-guided needle biopsy may be used to refine the diagnosis. Renal neoplasms have the potential to hemorrhage, resulting in hemoperitoneum that may produce a distended abdomen and a homogeneous fluid density with loss of organ contrast radiographically. Definitive diagnosis of hemoperitoneum is performed by abdominocentesis. Renal neoplasms generally present as cystic areas on ultrasound examination and may be mistaken for renal cysts, a more common and benign finding in many exotic mammals.

Primary renal tumors may be treated with nephrectomy and surgical excision (Fig. 14). In human patients, these tumors are often resistant to chemotherapy, and literature on chemotherapeutic use in domestic animals is rare. Ferret transitional cell carcinomas may respond to surgical excision,

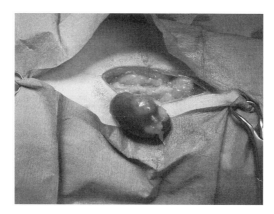

Fig. 14. This well-differentiated cystic papillary renal neoplasm (presumed adenoma) was found unilaterally on the left side. Nephrectomy was performed. No recurrence of neoplasia has occurred to date.

radiation therapy, and chemotherapy based on the location of the mass. A combination of doxorubicin and cyclophosphamide has been reported to prolong survival times in dogs, whereas cisplatin (50 mg/m^2 IV q 4 wks) has been reported to result in partial remission [31]. Mitoxantrone with or without piroxicam has shown some efficacy in dogs [31], but this efficacy has not been documented in small exotic mammals.

Metabolic disease

Rat chronic progressive nephrosis

Diagnosis of rat chronic progressive nephrosis (CPN) is based on clinical signs, isosthenuria, marked proteinuria, and an elevated BUN and creatinine consistent with renal insufficiency. Anemia, hyperphosphatemia, hypercholesterolemia, and hypoproteinemia may also be found on serum biochemical analysis. Affected rats may show evidence of polydipsia and polyuria, decreased appetite and weight loss, and diarrhea. Late-stage disease has been associated with hypertension and polyarteritis nodosa [18]. Physiologically, there are decreases in renal blood flow and glomerular filtration rate that must be considered when prescribing medication [32]. Differential diagnoses include chronic bacterial pyelonephritis, toxic nephrosis, congenital hydronephrosis, and ischemic injury.

Because of the chronic, debilitating nature of the disease, prognosis is poor. Treatment options include subcutaneous fluid therapy and dietary modification, which appears to play an important role in progression of CPN. Restricting calories, feeding diets low in protein (4% to 7%), substituting soy protein for casein, and substantially reducing caloric intake (low fat) may reduce the incidence and severity of CPN [33]. Studies have shown that omega-3 fatty acids have a number of beneficial effects on rat renal disease, including mitigating some of the detrimental effects of a high-fat diet and hyperlipidemia on glomerular function [34], attenuating the decline in glomerular filtration rate, the rise in blood pressure, and the proteinuria associated with renal disease [35], and maintaining significantly lower serum creatinine levels [36]. The primary rationale for the use of omega-3 fatty acids in renal disease is that they cause an alteration of eicosanoid metabolism, resulting in an increased production of vasodilatory compounds and a concurrent reduction of proinflammatory prostaglandins, leukotrienes, and thromboxanes [37]. Fish oils (docosohexanoic and eicosapentanoic acids), whole flaxseed, and flaxseed oil (alpha-linolenic acid) are rich sources of omega-3 fatty acids.

Other suggested supportive measures for general renal failure have included anabolic steroids and B complex vitamins to stimulate appetite and encourage red blood cell production, phosphorus binders, such as aluminum hydroxide, to limit dietary phosphorus absorption and control hyperphosphatemia and secondary renal hyperparathyroidism, and decreased salt intake to help diminish fluid loss and control high blood pressure.

Amyloidosis

Diagnosis is based on clinical signs, serum and urine analysis, and histopathology. Severe proteinuria and hypoalbuminemia are characteristic of significant glomerular disease, with elevations in BUN and creatinine occurring as renal failure ensues. In hamsters, a nephrotic syndrome is seen, whose clinical signs include ascites or subcutaneous edema concentrated in the ventral half of the body, hydrothorax, anorexia, and weight loss. Clinical pathology abnormalities in the hamster include hyperlipidemia (elevated cholesterol and triglycerides), hypoalbuminemia, and severe proteinuria.

Toxic nephropathies

Ferret ibuprofen toxicity

Diagnosis is based on known or presumed access to and ingestion of ibuprofen. Clinical signs are variable and nonspecific. Initial treatment for ibuprofen toxicosis depends on clinical signs, length of time from exposure, and quantity of the drug ingested. If the ferret is asymptomatic and ibuprofen ingestion is known to have occurred within 1 to 2 hours, gastrointestinal emesis may be induced using 3% hydrogen peroxide solution at 2.2 mL/kg. In symptomatic ferrets demonstrating signs that preclude emesis, gastric lavage may be performed in the anesthetized patient with a cuffed endotracheal tube in place. Activated charcoal absorbs ibuprofen and may be given at a dose of 1 to 3 g/kg [38]. Because of the enterohepatic recirculation of ibuprofen, dosing should be repeated [20]. An osmotic cathartic may be administered to facilitate removal of the activated charcoal-bound substance. Sorbitol at 3 mL/kg may be safely used with repeated charcoal administration [38]. When more severe clinical signs of toxicosis are present, treatment is primarily supportive and symptomatic. Stabilization is the first priority and may include oxygenation to treat brain hypoxia, diazepam or other anticonvulsants to control seizures, intravenous catheter placement for fluid diuresis, and thermoregulation. Gastrointestinal protectants include famotidine (0.5 mg/kg subcutaneously or intravenously) and sucralfate (125 mg PO every 6 hours). Prognosis is good with early and aggressive treatment.

Ferret zinc toxicosis

Clinical signs reported in zinc toxicosis include anorexia, lethargy, anemia, melena, diarrhea, and icterus [20]. Diagnosis is based on known exposure to zinc-containing products, radiographic evidence of heavy metals, clinical signs, and blood zinc levels. Treatment of zinc toxicity begins with efforts to remove zinc-containing materials by surgical extraction or by induced emesis or gastric lavage. Supportive therapy is essential and includes intravenous fluid therapy to maintain hydration status and induce diuresis, administration of gastrointestinal protectants (famotidine, sucralfate), and nutritional support. Continuous monitoring of the complete blood count (eg, packed cell volume, red blood cells), along with a serum chemistry panel (eg, BUN, creatinine, liver enzymes, electrolytes), is essential in assessing patient condition and response to therapy. Chelation therapy to enhance renal zinc excretion has been advocated by some individuals [39]. Considerations to take into account when deciding to use a chelation agent include the degree of serum zinc concentration, the clinical condition and hydration status of the patient, the degree of renal and gastrointestinal dysfunction, and the relative possibility of surgically removing an obvious zinc-containing object [39]. Calcium disodium ethylenediaminetetraacetic acid is the most commonly suggested chelation agent.

Special cases

Ferret Aleutian disease

A tentative diagnosis of Aleutian disease (AD) may be based on a combination of history, clinical signs, and hypergammaglobulinemia ($>20\%$ of the total protein showing a monoclonal gammopathy). Ferrets with total proteins greater than 7.5 g/dL, especially those with mildly decreased albumins and chronic weight loss, should be suspected of having AD. Anemia of chronic disease is seen in many cases and may be more severe in those involving hemorrhage secondary to platelet dysfunction, plasmacytic-lymphocytic bone marrow infiltration, or chronic renal failure. The white blood cell count is usually within normal limits, but it may show a lymphocyte-neutrophil reversal due to chronic systemic inflammation [40]. Azotemia and uremia are seen in late-stage disease.

Diagnosis of AD is confirmed ante mortem with a positive serum titer coupled with hypergammaglobulinemia or lymphoplasmacytic inflammation in tissue biopsy samples [41]. Two serologic tests are available for AD virus testing: the counterimmunoelectrophoresis (CEP or CIEP) test available from United Vaccines (Madison, Wisconsin) and the ELISA test for antibodies to the nonstructural proteins of the AD virus (available from Avecon Diagnostics, Bath, Pennsylvania). The ELISA test can be done on either blood or saliva. Unfortunately, the sensitivity and specificity of these two tests have been called into question. The University of Georgia DNA in situ Hybridization Laboratory tests serum for AD DNA using polymerase chain reaction (PCR) and for AD antibodies using CEP (antibody titers are reported out to 1:16,384, thus improving specificity). The DNA probe used for in situ hybridization was created using primers for the AD virus-G strain, and digoxigenin is used to label the DNA probes that are generated during the PCR reaction. This probe detects AD virus infection in mink, ferret, and skunk tissues. Thus the AD virus-G probe sequence is conserved sufficiently for detection of the AD virus across species (Kate E. Pennick, BS, Research Technician III and MS candidate, Veterinary Pathology, Athens, Georgia, personal communication, 2005). This laboratory can also test for AD virus DNA isolated from urine and feces to check for viral shedding.

No specific treatment exists for either the clinical disease or carrier state of AD in ferrets. Because the immune-mediated aspects of AD cause much of the glomerular pathology, immunosuppressive, anti-inflammatory therapy with prednisolone may help diminish clinical signs associated with glomerulonephritis. Other immunosuppressive drugs, such as azathioprine and cyclophosphamide, may help as well, but no controlled studies have been performed. Intravenous or subcutaneous fluid therapy may be needed to combat anorexia, dehydration, and uremia. Broad-spectrum antibiotics may be indicated when opportunistic bacterial infections occur as a result of parvovirus-associated leukopenia and immunosuppression. Feeding a high-calorie formulation by syringe is supportive.

The virus is susceptible to mechanical cleaning as well as phenol compounds, sodium hypochlorite, and quaternary ammonium products [42]. Quarantine in pet households is not practical because of the long incubation period in asymptomatic ferrets. Complete prevention would include strict sanitation, with isolation and culling of the AD-virus–seropositive ferrets. Culling of clinically normal, AD-positive ferrets is only recommended for breeding facilities and not for pet households.

Rabbit encephalitozoonosis

A definitive antemortem diagnosis of *Encephalitozoon cuniculi* is difficult because histopathology is required to demonstrate presence of the organism. Even post mortem, a definitive diagnosis of active *E cuniculi* infection may be difficult, because the organisms are not always visible. Affected kidneys may be grossly pitted and scarred and show histologic evidence of granulomatous inflammation. Granulomatous inflammatory response without presence of the organism indicates previous exposure, not necessarily active infection.

E cuniculi organisms may be found in the urine of infected laboratory rabbits; however, the organisms are shed intermittently and for only short periods (as long as 3 months) after infection, making urine testing impractical. PCR has been used positively to identify *E cuniculi* in encephalitozoon spores isolated in a primary tissue culture of the kidney from an encephalitozoonosis-suspected rabbit [43].

Because infection with *E cuniculi* is persistent in most cases, antibodies continue to be produced, and serologic testing may be a useful tool in rabbits showing signs suggestive of encephalitozoonosis. In the United States, Sound Diagnostics (Seattle, Washington) uses an ELISA to measure antibodies to the *E cuniculi* organisms. The amount of antibody is quantitated by optical density (OD) and compared with positive and negative controls. In the United Kingdom, an immunofluorescent antibody test is available that measures titers out to 1:132, thereby allowing for monitoring of treatment response (Jaime A. MacDonald, Associate of the Institute of BioMedical Science, personal communication, 2005). Negative titers indicate a lack of infection or early-stage infection when antibodies may be below the level of detection. The antibody response is initiated 3 to 4 weeks after infection and 4 weeks before histopathologic lesions are visible in the kidney or organisms are excreted in the urine. Lesions are not found in the brain until at least 8 weeks after first detectable antibody [44]. A positive titer with detection of antibodies does not differentiate between rabbits with an active infection, those with a latent infection, and those that developed an antibody response but are no longer infected. Positive results indicate previous exposure to the organism but do not confirm *E cuniculi* as a cause of disease. Follow-up samples may clarify equivocal results, because early-stage infection antibody levels will be considerably higher in the follow-up sample. Antibodies due to nonspecific reactivity or developed post infection will remain about the same. High levels of antibodies may be associated with disease, and antibody levels may decrease with time if infection is successfully eliminated, but months are usually required for this to occur. Using these guidelines, ELISAs may be useful in diagnosing infection and its association with clinical disease.

Treatment protocols for rabbits showing clinical signs suspicious for *E cuniculi* infection have been based on fundamental principles of therapy for granulomatous inflammation, on studies demonstrating efficacy against human encephalitozoon infections, and on in vitro susceptibility studies of *E cuniculi* organisms to various pharmacologic agents. It is difficult to assess the efficacy of therapeutic agents, because latent infections occur and some clinical cases may improve spontaneously without treatment, presumably as a result of the host's immune response [45]. In addition, clinical signs may not be associated with presence of the protozoa itself but rather with the inflammatory response that persists after the organism has been eliminated [46].

Several benzimidazole derivatives, including albendazole, oxibendazole, and fenbendazole, have been used to treat presumptive *E cuniculi* infections in rabbits. The use of albendazole is partially based on its effectiveness in treating and eliminating *Encephalitozoon* spp in human AIDS patients, along with its relief of clinical symptoms associated with infection [47]. One paper cites the efficacy of albendazole in reducing serum creatinine levels in rabbits experimentally infected with *E cuniculi* microsporidia [48]; however, the study did not measure creatinine levels in a group of non-treated control animals, nor did it perform histopathology to prove renal infection with the *E cuniculi* organism. Albendazole is embryotoxic and teratogenic in rabbits and has been associated with anecdotal reports of pancytopenia, fever, and death. Franssen and colleagues [49] demonstrated the in vitro efficacy of fumegillin, thiobendazole, oxibendazole, and albendazole in inhibiting *E cuniculi* proliferation in rabbit kidney tissue culture cells. In 2001, Suter and colleagues [50] described the potentially successful chemotherapeutic and prophylactic treatment of rabbit *E cuniculi* infections using fenbendazole. Administration of fenbendazole at 20 mg/kg daily for 30 days resulted in the apparent elimination of *E cuniculi* spores from the central nervous system of infected rabbits. Oxibendazole has been used against rabbit encephalitozoonosis with apparent safety, but definitive evidence of efficacy is lacking. Studies are ongoing at the University of California, Davis that may help clarify the confusing *E cuniculi* treatment picture. In vitro information suggests that albendazole and nitazoxamide (an equine antiprotozoal) can kill the organism and spare the host cell. In vivo studies on these two drugs, as well as itraconazole, are under way at this time (April 2005). Future in vitro and in vivo studies are planned for fenbendazole, ponazuril, and oxibendazole (Michelle Hawkins, DVM, Davis, California, personal communication, 2005).

An *E cuniculi* ELISA should be run on rabbits with azotemia and clinical signs of renal disease. Unfortunately, a positive titer does not confirm the association of renal disease with *E cuniculi* infection. Prognosis varies with degree of uremia and severity of clinical signs. Treatment for *E cuniculi* should be instituted based on the veterinarian's discretion and the patient's quality of life, along with supportive care in the form of fluid therapy, nutritional support, and medications to control hyperphosphatemia and gastrointestinal acidosis.

Summary

Various tools are used to diagnose renal disease in exotic mammals, including imaging techniques and urinary contrast studies, urinalysis, blood and serum chemical analysis, bacteriology, and serology. Treatment of the primary underlying cause may result in complete resolution of signs, as in cases of unilateral hydronephrosis, bacterial pyelonephritis, or obstructive urolithiasis. Renal insufficiency and renal failure are common sequelae to many diseases affecting the exotic mammal kidney, and in these cases fluid diuresis, treatment of secondary gastrointestinal signs and hyperphosphatemia, and general supportive care may improve the patient's quality of life for variable periods.

References

[1] Hoefer HL. Rabbit and ferret renal disease diagnosis. In: Fudge AM, editor. Laboratory medicine: avian and exotic pets. Philadelphia: WB Saunders; 2000. p. 311–8.
[2] Braun EJ. Comparative renal function in reptiles, birds, and mammals. Seminars in Avian and Exotic Pet Medicine 1998;7(2):2–71.

[3] Percy DH, Barthold SW. Gerbils. In: Pathology of laboratory rodents and rabbits. 2nd edition. Ames (IA): Blackwell Publishing; 2001. p. 197–208.

[4] Bihun C, Bauck L. Basic anatomy, physiology, husbandry, and clinical techniques. In: Quesenberry KE, Carpenter JW, editors. Ferrets, rabbits and rodents: clinical medicine and surgery. Philadelphia: WB Saunders; 2004. p. 286–98.

[5] Donnelly T. Basic anatomy, physiology, and husbandry (rabbits). In: Quesenberry KE, Carpenter JW, editors. Ferrets, rabbits and rodents: clinical medicine and surgery. Philadelphia: WB Saunders; 2004. p. 136–46.

[6] Grauer GF. Urinary tract disorders: renal failure. In: Nelson RW, Couto CG, editors. Small animal internal medicine. 3rd edition. St. Louis (MO): CV Mosby; 2003. p. 608–23.

[7] Benson KG, Paul-Murphy J. Clinical pathology of the domestic rabbit. Vet Clin North Am Exot Anim Pract 1999;2(3):539–51.

[8] Harkness JE, Wagner JE. Clinical procedures. In: The biology and medicine of rabbits and rodents. 4th edition. Baltimore (MD): Williams and Wilkins; 1995. p. 75–142.

[9] Esteves ML, Marini RP, Ryder EB, et al. Estimation of glomerular filtration rate and evaluation of renal function in ferrets (Mustela putorius furo). Am J Vet Res 1994;55(1):166–72.

[10] Antinoff N. Urinary disorders in ferrets. Seminars in Avian and Exotic Pet Medicine 1998; 7(2):89–92.

[11] Harcourt-Brown FM. Urogenital disease. In: Textbook of rabbit medicine. Oxford (UK): Butterworth Heinemann; 2002. p. 335–51.

[12] Saito K, Hosegawa A. Diseases and outcomes in rabbits with high BUN levels. J Vet Med Sci 2003;65(5):625–8.

[13] Morrisey JK, Ramer JC. Ferrets: clinical pathology and sample collection. Vet Clin North Am Exot Anim Pract 1999;2(3):553–64.

[14] Harcourt-Brown FM. Clinical pathology. In: Textbook of rabbit medicine. Oxford (UK): Butterworth Heinemann; 2002. p. 140–64.

[15] Sexauer CL, Matson JR. Anemia of chronic renal failure. Ann Clin Lab Sci 1981;11(6): 484–7.

[16] Tvedegaard E. Arterial disease in chronic renal failure—an experimental study in the rabbit. Acta Pathol Microbiol Immunol Scand Suppl 1987;290:1–28.

[17] Percy DH, Barthold SW. Mouse. In: Pathology of laboratory rodents and rabbits. Ames (IA): Blackwell Publishing; 2001. p. 3–106.

[18] Percy DH, Barthold SW. Rat. In: Pathology of laboratory rodents and rabbits. Ames (IA): Blackwell Publishing; 2001. p. 107–67.

[19] Knotek Z, Waldnerova L, Jekl V. Diagnostic urography of renal disorders in rats. Acta Vet Brno 2004;73:187–94.

[20] Orcutt CJ. Ferret urogenital diseases. Vet Clin North Am Exot Anim Pract 2003;6(1): 113–38.

[21] Carpenter JW. Exotic animal formulary. 3rd edition. St. Louis (MO): Elsevier Saunders; 2005.

[22] Nguyen HT, Moreland AF, Shields RP. Urolithiasis in ferrets (Mustela putorius). Lab Anim Sci 1979;5:243–5.

[23] Orcutt C. Treatment of urogenital disease in ferrets. Exotic DVM 2001;3(3):31–7.

[24] Tully T, Mitchell M, Heatley J. Urethral catheterization of male ferrets. Exotic DVM 2001; 3(2):29–31.

[25] Nolte DM, Carberry CA, Gannon KM, et al. Temporary tube cystostomy as a treatment for urinary obstruction secondary to adrenal disease in four ferrets. Journal of the American Animal Hospital Association 2002;38(6):527–32.

[26] Ross SJ, Osborne CA, Lulich JP, et al. Canine and feline nephrolithiasis, epidemiology, detection, and management. In: Osboren CA, Lulich JP, Bartges JW, editors. Vet Clin North Am Small Anim Pract 1999;29(1):231–50.

[27] Gahring DR, Crowe DT, Powers TE, et al. Comparative renal function studies of nephrotomy closure with and without sutures in dogs. J Am Vet Med Assoc 1977;171(6):537–41.

[28] Gaschen L, Ketz C, Lang J, et al. Ultrasonographic detection of adrenal gland tumor and uterolithiasis in a guinea pig. Vet Radiol Ultrasound 1998;39(1):43–6.

[29] Hoefer H. Guinea pig urolithiasis. Exotic DVM 2004;6(2):23–5.

[30] Pollock CG. Urogenital diseases. In: Quesenberry KE, Carpenter JW, editors. Ferrets, rabbits and rodents: clinical medicine and surgery. 2nd edition. Philadelphia: WB Saunders; 2003. p. 41–9.

[31] Ogilvie GK, Moore AS. Tumors of the urinary tract. In: Managing the veterinary cancer patient: a practice manual. Trenton (NJ): Veterinary Learning Systems; 1995. p. 402–11.

[32] Johnson-Delaney CA. Disease of the urinary system of commonly kept rodents: diagnosis and treatment. Seminars in Avian and Exotic Pet Medicine 1998;7(2):81–8.

[33] Donnelly TM. Diseases of small rodents. In: Quesenberry KE, Carpenter JW, editors. Ferrets, rabbits and rodents: clinical medicine and surgery. 2nd edition. Philadelphia: WB Saunders; 2003. p. 299–315.

[34] Lu J, Bankovic-Calic N, Ogborn M, et al. Detrimental effects of a high fat diet in early renal injury are ameliorated by fish oil in Han: SPRD-cy rats. J Nutr 2003;133:180–6.

[35] Ogborn MR, Nitschmann E, Bankovic-Calic N, et al. Dietary flax oil reduces renal injury, oxidized LDL content, and tissue n-6/n-3 FA ratio in experimental polycystic kidney disease. Lipids 2002;37(11):1059–65.

[36] Ingram AJ, Parbtani A, Clark WF, et al. Effects of flaxseed and flax oil diets in a rat-5/6 renal ablation model. Am J Kidney Dis 1995;25(2):320–9.

[37] Plotnick AN. The role of omega-3 fatty acids in renal disorders. J Am Vet Med Assoc 1996; 209(1):906–10.

[38] Richardson JA, Balabuszko RA. Managing ferret toxicosis. Exotic DVM 2000;2(4):23–6.

[39] Talcott PA. Zinc poisoning. In: Peterson ME, Talcott PA, editors. Small animal toxicology. Philadelphia: WB Saunders; 2001. p. 756–61.

[40] Williams B. Infectious diseases: Aleutian disease. Management of the ferret for veterinary professionals: proceedings. Vol. 2. 2000. p. 69–70.

[41] Langlois I. Viral diseases in ferrets. Vet Clin North Am Exot Anim Pract 2005;8(1):139–60.

[42] Fox JG, Pearson CP, Gorham R. Viral diseases. In: Fox JG, editor. Biology and diseases of the ferret. Baltimore (MD): Williams and Wilkins; 1998. p. 360–6.

[43] Furuya K, Kukui D, et al. Isolation of Encephalitozoon cuniculi using primary tissue culture techniques from a rabbit colony showing encephalitozoonosis. Vet Med Sci 2001;63(2): 203–6.

[44] Cox JC, Gallichio HA. Serological and histological studies on adult rabbits with recent, naturally acquired encephalitozoonosis. Res Vet Sci 1978;24(2):260–1.

[45] Harcourt-Brown FM. Infectious diseases of domestic rabbits. In: Textbook of rabbit medicine. Oxford (UK): Butterworth Heinemann; 2002. p. 361–85.

[46] Harcourt-Brown FM. Encephalitozoon cuniculi in pet rabbits. Vet Rec 2003;152:427–31.

[47] De Groote MA, Visvesvara G, et al. Polymerase chain reaction and culture confirmation of disseminated Encephalitozoon cuniculi in a patient with AIDS: successful therapy with albendazole. J Infect Dis 1995;171:1375–8.

[48] Conkova E, Cellarova E, Neuschl J, et al. The dynamics of creatinine and urea concentrations in the blood serum of rabbits infected by Encephalitozoon cuniculi microsporidium and treated with albendazole. Acta Vet (Beogr) 1999;49(5–6):321–6.

[49] Franssen FFJ, Lumeij JT, Van Knapen F. Susceptibility of Encephalitozoon cuniculi to several drugs in vitro. Antimicrob Agents Chemother 1995;39:1265–8.

[50] Suter C, Muller-Doblies UU, Hatt J-M, et al. Prevention and treatment of Encephalitozoon cuniculi infection in rabbits with fenbendazole. Vet Rec 2001;148:478–80.

VETERINARY
CLINICS
Exotic Animal Practice

Vet Clin Exot Anim 9 (2006) 97–106

ELSEVIER
SAUNDERS

Types of Renal Disease in Avian Species

Robert E. Schmidt, DVM, PhD, DABVP

Zoo/Exotic Pathology Service, PO Box 267, Greenview, CA 96037, USA

Renal disease in birds is frequently encountered. Like most other animals, birds are susceptible to a full spectrum of renal insults, such as toxins, tumors, infections, and degenerative conditions. Accurate diagnosis of renal disease is based on a complete history, physical examination, and laboratory evaluation of the patient. Because it is often required for a more definitive diagnosis, special attention is given to histopathologic evaluation of renal tissue, whether through a premortem biopsy or collection at gross necropsy.

Congenital disease

Although not frequently reported, congenital renal lesions are occasionally seen in birds [1]. Renal hypoplasia or aplasia occurs sporadically in birds. It is usually diagnosed as an incidental necropsy finding. Divisional aplasia is common in some breeds of chickens. The cranial division is most likely to be absent. Compensatory hypertrophy of the opposite kidney is generally present.

Renal cysts may be solitary or multiple. If the lesion is severe, the result will be renal failure. Glomerular hypervascularity has been reported in canaries [2]. It leads to glomerular deformation but does not result in immediate renal failure.

Infectious disease

Bacterial

Bacteria can enter the kidney either by ascending the ureters or by hematogenous spread. In either type of infection, the kidneys may be grossly enlarged with variable degrees of necrosis. Histologic lesions suggestive of bacterial nephritis include tubular dilatation and impaction with inflammatory cells [3]. Acute ascending infections are characterized by abundant

---

E-mail address: zooexotic@sisqtel.net

bacteria found in tubules and occasionally in the interstitium. As nephritis becomes chronic, tubular necrosis, cyst formation, distortion, and interstitial fibrosis with mononuclear cell infiltration become evident. Initial hematogenous lesions may be present in glomeruli. Organisms associated with necrosis and a pleocellular inflammatory infiltrate may be seen.

Necrosis of the tubular epithelium is sometimes prominent, but inflammation may be minimal or nonexistent in cases of bacterial nephritis. Distal collecting tubules and cortical collecting ducts are primarily affected by bacterial infections. Subacute ascending infections have a marked inflammatory response with heterophils in the lumen of the tubules. Tubulointerstitial lesions are locally extensive. With severe locally extensive lesions, it may be difficult to determine whether the infection began in the tubules and involved the interstitium or vice versa.

A wide range of gram-positive and gram-negative bacteria are known to cause kidney disease, either as an ascending infection or as part of a systemic disease. Staphylococci and streptococci are common pathogens [4,5]. Other bacteria that can affect the kidney include members of Enterobacteriaceae, *Listeria* sp, *Erysipelothrix rhusiophathiae*, and *Pasteurella* sp [6].

Mycobacterial and *Chlamydophila psittaci* infections are generally systemic infections. They may cause lesions in the kidney [7] but often do not. Mycobacterial lesions are similar to those found in other tissues. Renal lesions caused by *C psittaci* are characterized by interstitial inflammation composed primarily of histiocytes, plasma cells, and lymphocytes, with intracytoplasmic organisms seen in histiocytes in some cases. Any bacterial organism associated with sepsis may be found in avian renal tissue.

Mycotic

Fungal infection of the kidney occurs either as an extension of a fungal infection of the abdominal air sacs [8,9] or as a component of fungemia where a fungus has invaded a vessel, resulting in fungal thrombosis of blood vessels. Fungal hyphae in the lesion give it specificity.

Parasitic—protozoal

Isospora sp and *Eimeria* sp are found in the kidneys of nearly all species of wild ducks and geese [10–14], as well as in other avian species [15–17]. Organisms are predominantly found in the epithelium of perilobular collecting ducts and the medullary collecting tract. *Eimeria truncata* may cause a more severe disease in juvenile waterfowl. Organisms are found in tubular epithelial cells or free in the lumen associated with inflammatory cells and necrotic debris.

Cryptosporidial infection of the kidney of birds is reported [18–21]. Kidneys appear swollen and pale. Slight proliferation of tubular epithelial cells may be seen, and organisms are present on their surface.

Encephalitozoon hellem is a potential cause of renal disease. Lesions are most commonly seen in lovebirds and budgerigars but have been reported in other psittacine birds [22,23]. Gross changes may be absent, or small pale foci may be present in the renal parenchyma. Histologically, small protozoal organisms are present in cells and may be free in necrotic foci and the lumen of the renal tubules.

Systemic sarcosporidial infection may lead to interstitial nephritis with an infiltrate that is primarily lymphoplasmacytic [24]. Organisms are usually not seen. Schizonts of leukocytozoon can also be found in the kidney [25].

Parasitic—metazoal

Trematodes may be incidental findings or lead to clinical renal disease in some birds. These infections are most common in waterfowl. The flukes are found in collecting tubules in the medullary cone [26,27]. Severe infections result in obstruction of the tubules, variable inflammation and necrosis, and secondary dilatation proximal to the obstruction.

Visceral larval migrans due to *Baylisascaris procyonis* may lead to necrotic tracts and larvae within the kidneys [28].

Viral

Adenovirus infection of the kidney is seen in a variety of birds [29,30]. Grossly there may be some nonspecific renal enlargement. Microscopic lesions are usually minimal, ranging from mild interstitial mononuclear cell infiltration to tubular epithelial cell vacuolation and necrosis. Scattered tubular epithelial cells have karyomegalic nuclei containing large, darkly eosinophilic or basophilic inclusion bodies.

Polyomavirus infection may be acute and cause the kidneys to be slightly swollen. Virus may be recovered from the kidney [31]. Histologically, renal tubular epithelial cells may have karyomegaly, with affected nuclei containing clear or amophophilic, slightly granular inclusion bodies. These may be differentiated from those of adenovirus by their tinctorial properties.

Both primary and secondary lesions may occur in nonbudgerigar psittacine birds with avian polyomavirus disease [32,33]. Intranuclear inclusion bodies and accompanying karyomegaly are commonly seen in mesangial cells. Glomeruli will appear swollen. As many as 70% of these birds will develop a secondary glomerulopathy. This lesion is caused by the deposition of dense aggregates of immune complexes.

Finches with polyomavirus infection may have both renal tubular epithelial and mesangial karyomegaly with intranuclear inclusion bodies.

Nonsuppurative inflammation may be present in the renal interstitium in other viral infections, including reovirus [34] and paramyxovirus [35,36]. Paramyxovirus-1 in pigeons may cause an interstitial lymphoplasmacytic nephritis and tubular necrosis, with granular and hyaline casts present in the tubules. West Nile virus causes a variable lymphocytic interstitial nephritis as part of generalized disease [37].

Other viruses that may cause renal disease include coronavirus, togavirus, and influenza A virus [38].

Inflammatory disease of undetermined cause

Except as a sequela to polyomavirus infection (discussed in the previous section), immune complex glomerulopathies are infrequently documented in birds, but autoimmune glomerulonephritis has been produced [39–41]. In chronic cases, there may be proliferation of parietal epithelium and glomerular crescent formation. Eventually glomerular shrinkage, fibrous connective tissue proliferation, and sclerosis occur.

Noninfectious disease

Avian renal disease has a wide variety of noninfectious causes. Many of these result in chronic disease with a common gross and histologic appearance.

Dehydration results in reduced urine flow and sludging of the urate crystals within the tubules. Gross lesions are characterized by multifocal white to yellow-white foci or streaks that represent urate deposits. The gross appearance is similar to that of mineralization. Microscopically, urates are dissolved during the fixation process but leave behind needle-shaped and amorphous spaces surrounded by an eosinophilic protein matrix [42,43].

Disorders of protein metabolism may lead to elevation of uric acid; however, whether this in turn may result in urate deposition has not been established [44–46].

Other nutritional problems may result in renal disease. Metastatic mineralization of the kidney is a common lesion in nestling parrots and to a lesser extent in adult birds. A nutritional imbalance is suspected. Renal lipidosis may be secondary to a high-fat diet or chronic hepatic disease. On a gross level the kidneys are pale, and microscopically there is fat in tubular epithelial cells. Lipid-containing macrophages are usually present in glomerular capillaries. Vitamin A deficiency leads to squamous metaplasia of the epithelium of the ureters and collecting ducts, which in advanced cases results in the transformation of the ureteral epithelium to a keratinized epithelium [25,47–51]. High-cholesterol diets have also been associated with diffuse renal disease, including proliferative glomerulopathy, periglomerular fibrosis, multifocal interstitial nephritis, and lipid-laden cells within the glomeruli of pigeons [52].

Renal amyloidosis is most frequently observed in waterfowl and small passerine birds. Multiple organs in addition to the kidney are generally involved. Grossly the kidneys may be enlarged, pale, and somewhat friable. Histologically, the amyloid is eosinophilic or amphophilic and may be deposited in glomerular or tubular basement membranes and the walls of renal arteries and arterioles [25,53,54].

Iron storage disease primarily affects the liver, but iron pigment is also seen in renal tubular cells in many affected birds. The iron does not cause an inflammatory or degenerative response [25,55].

Renal disease and lesion formation may be secondary to a wide variety of conditions [56–59]. Ischemic (hemoglobinuric, myoglobinuric) nephrosis is secondary to a number of problems. Hemoglobinuric nephrosis is infrequent because of the rarity of hemolytic disease in birds. Myoglobinuric nephrosis may be a sequela to exertional rhabdomyolysis or severe crushing injury to muscle [60]. In both cases, the kidneys may be dark brown. Tubular degeneration and lumenal accumulation of amorphous eosinophilic material resembling myoglobin are seen microscopically in proximal convoluted tubules, and eosinophilic casts are noted in collecting tubules.

Toxic nephropathies

History is important in making a diagnosis of toxic nephropathy, because most renal toxins cause similar gross and histologic lesions; therefore, a definitive causative diagnosis is often not possible based on gross and histopathologic changes alone. Sometimes the tentative diagnosis is made by excluding all other possibilities [61].

Vitamin D_3– and vitamin D_3 analogue–based rodenticides are toxic in birds. These rodenticides cause increased intestinal absorption of calcium and hypercalcemia. Decreased urinary calcium excretion may also occur. Calcium is deposited in soft tissues, including the kidney [25].

Gentamicin sulfate and amikacin are two aminoglycoside antibiotics that are commonly used in birds. Gentamicin sulfate is more nephrotoxic than amikacin. Aminoglycoside toxicity results in kidney enlargement and changes resembling those seen with other causes of renal failure [62].

Lead and zinc toxicity both may cause acute tubular necrosis [63–67]. Gross changes vary from none to swollen, pale kidneys. Cadmium, mercury, and arsenic are also nephrotoxic [25].

Several mycotoxins, including oosporein, citrinin, and ochratoxin, have been shown to cause disease in poultry or domestic waterfowl [68–70]. Aflatoxins may also be a problem; they can cause degeneration of the proximal convoluted tubules and thickening of glomerular basement membranes [25,71].

Excessive salt ingestion leads to renal problems that result in urate deposition and gross and histologic lesions [72,73].

A variety of other nephrotoxins have been reported to affect birds [61,66,74,75].

Physical/other nephropathies

Acute renal hypoxia/ischemia is usually related to a localized or generalized vascular problem. The results are tubular necrosis, protein leakage, and urate deposition. Lesions are similar to the various problems discussed under metabolic disorders, and differential diagnoses include many of these conditions. Renal hemorrhage may be secondary to trauma, ischemia, or a variety of primary disease conditions. The hemorrhage may be visible grossly and may affect both interstitium and tubules. The end result of many of these conditions is chronic or end-stage renal disease with severe fibrosis [25].

Neoplastic disease

Renal tumors are reported in many species of birds but are particularly common in the budgerigar [76–78]. Renal carcinoma is the most common tumor of the kidney; however, adenoma, nephroblastoma, cystadenoma, fibrosarcoma, lymphosarcoma, and other neoplasms are also reported in the avian kidney [25].

The most common presenting sign of renal neoplasia is unilateral or bilateral lameness or paralysis [79]. These symptoms result from compression of the lumbar and sacral nerve plexi as they pass through or dorsal to the kidney, respectively, or from tumor growth into and adjacent to the synsacrum. Skeletal muscle atrophy and osteopenia may also be seen. Metastasis is occasionally reported [80].

Embryonal nephromas (nephroblastomas) are most commonly reported in chickens but are also found in psittacine and small passerine birds. They are usually unilateral but may be bilateral and are grossly similar to carcinomas [25].

Lymphosarcoma may be isolated to the kidney but is usually a part of generalized neoplastic disease. Grossly, the kidneys are pale, mottled, and moderately firm with nodular or diffuse cell infiltration. Myeloproliferative disease and histiocytosis are also reported in the avian kidney [81–83].

Other primary sarcomas are possible but are rarely reported, and metastatic sarcomas are infrequent. Malignant melanoma may affect the kidney, usually as a part of multicentric neoplastic proliferation [25].

References

[1] Tudor DC. Congenital defects of poultry. Worlds Poult Sci J 1979;35:20–6.
[2] Zwart P, Vroege C, Boostsma R, et al. Glomerular hypervascularity. A congenital defect in a canary (*Serinus canarius*). Avian Pathol 1974;3:59–60.
[3] Siller WG. Renal pathology of the fowl—a review. Avian Pathol 1981;10:187–262.
[4] Bounous DI, Schaeffer DO, Roy A. Coagulase-negative *Staphylococcus* sp. septicemia in a love-bird. J Am Vet Med Assoc 1989;195:1120–2.

[5] Gevaert D, Nelis J, Verhaeghe B. Plasma chemistry and urine analysis in Salmonella-induced polyuria in racing pigeons (Columbia livia). Avian Pathol 1991;20:379–86.

[6] Shibatani M, Suzuki T, Chujo M, et al. Disseminated intravascular coagulation in chickens inoculated with Erysipelothrix rhusiopathiae. J Comp Pathol 1997;117:147–56.

[7] Sato Y, Aoyagi T, Matsuura S. An occurrence of avian tuberculosis in hooded merganser (Lophodytes cucullatus). Avian Dis 1996;40:941–4.

[8] Phalen DN, Ambrus S, Graham DL. The avian urinary system: form, function, diseases. Presented at the Annual Conference of the Association of Avian Veterinarians. New Orleans, LA, 1990.

[9] Tham VL, Purcell DA, Schultz DJ. Fungal nephritis in a grey-headed albatross. J Wildl Dis 1974;10:306–9.

[10] Page CD, Haddad K. Coccidial infections in birds. Seminars in Avian and Exotic Pet Medicine 1995;4:136–44.

[11] Wobeser G. Renal coccidiosis in mallard and pintail ducks. J Wildl Dis 1974;10:249–55.

[12] Oksanen A. Mortality associated with renal coccidiosis in juvenile wild greylag geese (Anser anser anser). J Wildl Dis 1994;30(4):554–6.

[13] Gajadhar AA, Cawthorn RJ, Rainnie DJ. Experimental studies on the life cycle of a renal coccidium of lesser snow geese (Anser c. caerulescens). Can J Zool 1982;60:2085–92.

[14] Gajadhar AA, Cawthorn RJ, Wobeser GA. Prevalence of renal coccidia in wild waterfowl in Saskatchewan. Can J Zool 1983;61:2631–3.

[15] Montgomery RD, Novilla MN, Shillinger RB. Renal coccidiosis caused by Eimeria gavial sp. n. in a common loon (Gavia immer). Avian Dis 1978;22:809–14.

[16] Leighton FA, Gajadhar AA. Eimeria fraterculae sp. n. in the kidneys of Atlantic puffins (Fratercula arctica) from Newfoundland, Canada: species description and lesions. J Wildl Dis 1986;22(4):520–6.

[17] Gajadhar AA, Leighton FA. Eimeria wobeseri sp. n. and Eimeria goelandi sp. n. (Protozoa: Apicomplexa) in the kidneys of herring gulls (Larus argentatus). J Wildl Dis 1988;24(3):538–46.

[18] Trampel DW, Pepper TM, Blagburn BL. Urinary tract cryptosporidiosis in commercial laying hens. Avian Dis 2000;44:479–84.

[19] Randall CJ. Renal and nasal cryptosporidiosis in a junglefowl (Gallus sonneratii). Vet Rec 1986;119:130–1.

[20] Nakamura K, Abe F. Respiratory (especially pulmonary) and urinary infections of Cryptosporidium in layer chickens. Avian Pathol 1988;17:703–11.

[21] Gardiner CH, Imes GD. Cryptosporidium sp. in the kidneys of a black-throated finch. J Am Vet Med Assoc 1984;185(11):1401–2.

[22] Poonacha KB, William PD, Stamper RD. Encephalitizoonosis in a parrot. J Am Vet Med Assoc 1985;186(7):700–2.

[23] Pulparampil N, Graham D, Phalen D. Encephalitozoon hellem in two eclectus parrots (Eclectus roratus): identification from archival tissues. J Eukaryot Microbiol 1998;45(6):651–5.

[24] Smith JH, Neill PJG, Dillard EA. Pathology of experimental Sarcocystis falcatula infections of canaries (Serinus canarius) and pigeons (Columba livia). J Parasitol 1990;76(1):59–68.

[25] Schmidt RE, Reavill DR, Phalen D. Pathology of pet and aviary birds. Ames (IA): Iowa State Press: Blackwell Publishing; 2003.

[26] Schmidt RE, Hubbard GB. Urinary system. In: Atlas of zoo animal pathology, Vol. II. Boca Raton (FL): CRC Press; 1987. p. 83–96.

[27] Stunkard HW. Renicolid trematodes (Digenea) from the renal tubules of birds. Ann Parasitol Hum Comp 1971;46:109–18.

[28] Evans RH. Baylisascaris procyonis (Nematoda: Ascarididae) larva migrans in free-ranging wildlife in Orange County, California. J Parasitol 2002;88(2):299–301.

[29] Mori F, Touchi A, Suwa T, et al. Inclusion bodies containing adenovirus-like particles in the kidneys of psittacine birds. Avian Pathol 1989;18:197–202.

[30] Cheng AC, Wang MS, Chen XY, et al. Pathologic and pathological characteristics of new type gosling viral enteritis first observed in China. World J Gastroenterol 2001;7(5):678–84.

[31] Guerin J, Gelfi J, Dubois L. A novel polyomavirus (goose hemorrhagic polyomavirus) is the agent of hemorrhagic nephritis enteritis of geese. J Virol 2000;74:4523–9.

[32] Gerlach H, Enders F, Casares M, et al. Membranous glomerulopathy as an indicator of avian polyomavirus infection in Psittaciformes. J Avian Med Surg 1998;12:248–54.

[33] Phalen DN, Wilson VG, Graham DL. Characterization of the avian polyomavirus–associated glomerulopathy of nestling parrots. Avian Dis 1996;40:140–9.

[34] Ni Y, Kemp MC. A comparative study of avian reovirus pathogenicity: virus spread and replication and induction of lesions. Avian Dis 1995;39:554–66.

[35] Barton JT, Bickford AA, Cooper GL, et al. Avian paramyxovirus type 1 infections in racing pigeons in California. I. Clinical signs, pathology, and serology. Avian Dis 1992;36:463–8.

[36] Cross G. Paramyxovirus-1 infection (Newcastle disease) of pigeons. Seminars in Avian and Exotic Pet Medicine 1995;4:92–5.

[37] Kramer LD, Bernard KA. West Nile virus infection in birds and mammals. Ann N Y Acad Sci 2001;951:84–93.

[38] Ritchie BW, editor. Avian viruses: function and control. Lake Worth (FL): Wingers Publishing; 1995.

[39] Tucker FL, Strugill BC, Bolton WK. Ultrastructural studies of experimental autoimmune glomerulonephritis in normal and bursectomized chickens. Lab Invest 1985;53:563–70.

[40] Bolton WK, Tucker FL, Sturgill BC. Experimental autoimmune glomerulonephritis in chickens. J Clin Lab Immunol 1980;3:179–84.

[41] Bolton WK, Tucker FL, Sturgill BC. New avian model of experimental glomerulonephritis consistent with mediation by cellular immunity. Nonhumorally mediated glomerulonephritis in chickens. J Clin Invest 1984;73:1263–76.

[42] Lumeij JT. Plasma urea, creatinine and uric acid concentrations in response to dehydration in racing pigeons. Avian Pathol 1987;16:377–82.

[43] Julian R. Water deprivation as a cause of renal disease of chickens. Avian Pathol 1982;11:615–7.

[44] Angel R, Ballam G. Dietary protein effect on parakeet plasma uric acid, reproduction, and growth. Presented at the Annual Conference of the Association of Avian Veterinarians. Philadelphia, PA, 1995.

[45] Chandra M. Hematologic changes in nephritis in poultry induced by diets high in protein, high in calcium, containing urea, or deficient in vitamin A. Poult Sci 1984;63:710–6.

[46] McNabb FMA, McNabb RA, Steeves HR. Renal mucoid materials in pigeons fed high and low protein diets. Auk 1973;90:14–8.

[47] Forbes NA, Cooper JE. Fatty liver–kidney syndrome of merlins. In: Redig PT, Cooper JE, Remple D, et al, editors. Raptor biomedicine. Minneapolis (MN): University of Minnesota Press; 1993. p. 45–8.

[48] Harper EJ, Skinner ND. Clinical nutrition of small psittacines and passerines. Seminars in Avian and Exotic Pet Medicine 1998;7:116–27.

[49] Kolmstetter CM, Ramsay EC. Effects of feeding on plasma uric acid and urea concentrations in blackfooted penguins (*Spheniscus demersus*). J Avian Med Surg 2000;14(3):177–9.

[50] Whitehead CC, Siller WG. Experimentally induced fatty liver and kidney syndrome in the young turkey. Res Vet Sci 1983;34:73–6.

[51] Schoemaker NJ, Lumeij JT, Beynen AC. Polyuria and polydypsia due to vitamin and mineral oversupplementation of the diet of a salmon crested cockatoo (*Cacatua moluccensis*) and blue and gold macaw (*Ara ararauna*). Avian Pathol 1997;26:201–9.

[52] Klumpp SA, Wagner WD. Survey of the pathologic findings in a large production colony of pigeons, with special reference to pseudomembranous stomatitis and nephritis. Avian Dis 1986;30:740–50.

[53] Nakamura K, Tanaka H, Kodama Y, et al. Systemic amyloidosis in laying Japanese quail. Avian Dis 1998;42:209–14.

[54] Rigdon RH. Occurrence and association of amyloid with diseases in birds and mammals including man: a review. Tex Rep Biol Med 1974;32:665–82.

[55] Brayton C. Amyloidosis, hemochromatosis, and atherosclerosis in a roseate flamingo (*Phoenicopterus ruber*). Ann N Y Acad Sci 1992;653:184–90.

[56] Forman MF, Wideman RF. Renal responses of normal and preascitic broilers to systemic hypotension induced by unilateral pulmonary artery occlusion. Poult Sci 1999;78:1773–85.

[57] Frank RK, Newman J, Ruth GR. Lesions of perirenal hemorrhage syndrome in growing turkeys. Avian Dis 1991;35:523–34.

[58] Larochelle D, Morin M, Bernier G. Sudden death in turkeys with perirenal hemorrhage: pathological observations and possible pathogenesis of the disease. Avian Dis 1992;36: 114–24.

[59] Wideman RF, Laverty G. Kidney function in domestic fowl with chronic occlusion of the ureter and caudal renal veins. Poult Sci 1986;65:2148–55.

[60] Bermudez AJ, Hopkins BA. Hemoglobinuric nephrosis in a rhea (*Rhea americana*). Avian Dis 1995;39:661–5.

[61] LaBonde J. Toxicity in pet avian patients. Seminars in Avian and Exotic Pet Medicine 1995; 4(1):23–31.

[62] Flammer K, Clark CH, Drewes LA, et al. Adverse effects of gentamycin in scarlet macaws and galahs. Am J Vet Res 1990;51:404–7.

[63] Bailey TA, Samour JH, Naldo J, et al. Lead toxicosis in captive houbara bustards (Chlamydotis undulata maqueenii). Vet Rec 1995;137:193–4.

[64] Brown C, Wallner-Pendleton E, Armstrong D. Lead poisoning in captive gentoo penguins (*Pygoscelis papua papua*). Presented at the Annual Conference of the American Association of Zoo Veterinarians. Omaha, NE, 1996. p. 298–301.

[65] Mateo R, Dolz JC, Aguilar Serrano JM, et al. An epizootic of lead poisoning in greater flamingos (*Phoenicopterus ruber roseus*) in Spain. J Wildl Dis 1997;33(1):131–4.

[66] Degernes LA. Toxicities in waterfowl. Seminars in Avian and Exotic Pet Medicine 1995;4(1): 15–22.

[67] Holz P, Phelan J, Slocombe R, et al. Zinc toxicosis as a cause of sudden death in orange-bellied parrots (*Neophema chrysogaster*). J Avian Med Surg 2000;14:37–41.

[68] Manning RO, Wyatt RD. Toxicity of *Aspergillus ochraceus* contaminated wheat and different chemical forms of ochratoxin A in broiler chicks. Poult Sci 1984;63:458–65.

[69] Pegram RA, Wyatt RD. Avian gout caused by oosporein, a mycotoxin produced by *Chaetomium trilaterale*. Poult Sci 1982;60:2429–40.

[70] Pegram RA, Wyatt RD, Smith TL. Oosporein toxicosis in the turkey poult. Avian Dis 1982; 26:47–59.

[71] Mollenhauer HH, Corrier DE, Huff WE, et al. Ultrastructure of hepatic and renal lesions in chickens fed aflatoxin. Am J Vet Res 1989;50:771–7.

[72] Bennett DC, Bowes VA, Hughes MR, et al. Suspected sodium toxicity in hand-reared great blue heron (*Ardea herodia*) chicks. Avian Dis 1992;36:743–8.

[73] Wages DP, Ficken MD, Cook ME, et al. Salt toxicosis in commercial turkeys. Avian Dis 1995;39:158–61.

[74] Sarkar K, Narbaitz R, Pokrupa R, et al. The ultrastructure of nephrocalcinosis induced in chicks by *Cestrum diurnum* leaves. Vet Pathol 1981;18:62–70.

[75] Morgulis MS, Oliveira GH, Dagli ML, et al. Acute 2,4-dichlorophenoxyacetic acid intoxication in broiler chicks. Poult Sci 1998;77:509–15.

[76] Macwhirter P, Pyke D, Wayne J. Use of carboplatin in the treatment of renal adenocarcinoma in a budgerigar. Exotic DVM Veterinary Magazine 2002;4(2):11–2.

[77] Neuman U, Kummerfeld N. Neoplasms in budgerigars (*Melopsittacus undulatus*): clinical, pathomorphological and serological findings with special consideration of kidney tumours. Avian Pathol 1983;12:353–62.

[78] Van Toor AJ, Zwart P, Kaal G. Adenocarcinoma of the kidney in two budgerigars. Avian Pathol 1984;13:145–50.

[79] Freeman KP, Hahn KA, Jones MP, et al. Right leg muscle atrophy and osteopenia caused by renal adenocarcinoma in a cockatiel (*Melopsittacus undulatus*). Vet Radiol Ultrasound 1999; 40(2):144–7.

[80] Latimer KS, Ritchie BW, Campagnoli RP, et al. Metastatic renal carcinoma in an African grey parrot (*Psittacus erithacus erithacus*). J Vet Diagn Invest 1996;8:261–4.

[81] Coleman CW, Oliver R. Lymphosarcoma in a juvenile blue and gold macaw (*Ara araruana*) and a mature canary (*Seriunus canaries*). Journal of the Association of Avian Veterinarians 1994;8:64–8.

[82] Hafner S, Goodwin MA, Smith EJ, et al. Multicentric histiocytosis in young chickens. Gross and light microscopic pathology. Avian Dis 1996;40:202–9.

[83] Schmidt RE. Morphologic diagnosis of avian neoplasms. Seminars in Avian and Exotic Pet Medicine 1992;1:73–9.

VETERINARY
CLINICS
Exotic Animal Practice

Vet Clin Exot Anim 9 (2006) 107–128

Diagnosis and Treatment of Avian Renal Disease

Christal Pollock, DVM, DABVP-Avian

*College of Veterinary Medicine, Kansas State University, 1800 Denison Avenue,
Manhattan, KS 66502, USA*

Significant causes of renal disease in the companion parrot include dehydration, hypovitaminosis A, excessive dietary vitamin D_3, heavy metal toxicity, bacterial nephritis secondary to systemic disease, and renal carcinoma. Additional important differentials include renal lipidosis in merlins and amyloidosis in waterfowl and songbirds. Diagnosis of renal disease may rely on the identification of consistent clinical signs, clinical pathology, survey radiographs, and laparoscopic evaluation and biopsy of the kidneys. Treatment of avian renal disease relies on supportive care such as fluid therapy and nutritional support. Other treatments vary with the underlying cause and the clinical picture but may include systemic antibiotics, diuretics, parenteral vitamin A, and agents to lower uric acid levels such as allopurinol. Reports on the incidence of renal disease in the avian patient vary, but renal disease is common in poultry and birds of prey [1,2]. Clinical renal disease is probably under-recognized in the companion bird, with the notable exception of renal tumors in the budgerigar (*Melopsittacus undulatus*).

Clinical signs of renal disease

Vague clinical signs such as weakness, anorexia, vomiting, or regurgitation often predominate in avian renal disease [3,4]. Early signs of mechanical compression or invasion of spinal nerves may include twitching and subtle signs of pain [3–8]. In rare instances, painful behavior may include feather picking or self-mutilation over the synsacrum [4,8,9]. As disease progresses, hematuria, unilateral or bilateral limb paresis, and disuse muscle atrophy may be observed [3,4,10,11]. Renomegaly may also lead to

E-mail address: cpollock@vet.k-state.edu

doi:10.1016/j.cvex.2005.10.007

cloacal atony and constipation [4,7]. Metabolic abnormalities, particularly those caused by bacterial or viral nephritis, may cause persistent polydipsia/polyuria and, less commonly, oliguria, anuria, or seizure activity [3,4,6,8].

Important differentials for primary renal disease

Metabolic causes of renal disease

Dehydration is an important contributor to renal disease. Severe or persistent dehydration increases resorption of water causing a subsequent reduction in urine flow. As uric acid secretion decreases, urates may precipitate in renal tubules and ureters leading to impaction and potentially renal failure [2,12–15].

Deposition of lipid in renal tubules is an important problem of chicks, poults, and adult captive merlins (*Falco columbarius*) [16,17]. This condition has also been reported in the budgerigar parakeet and sulfur-crested cockatoo (*Cacatua galerita*) [7]. Renal lipidosis has been correlated with high-fat or low-protein diets, starvation, biotin deficiency, and chronic liver disease [2,15–17]. Poultry may exhibit acute onset of lethargy, followed by paralysis and death [16,17]. Merlins generally die acutely and are found in good flesh or slightly overweight [16].

Neoplasia of the avian kidney

In a study of 1203 budgerigar parakeets, 16% had tumors, and 23% of these tumors were renal [11]. The most common tumor in the bird is renal adenocarcinoma, which sometimes causes osteolysis and sclerosis of the ileum and synsacrum and potentially infiltrates nearby muscle and other surrounding tissue [7,15]. Distant metastasis to the skin, lung, liver, and oviduct is rare [15,18–20].

Nutritional causes of renal disease

Excess dietary protein or calcium, hypovitaminosis A, or hypervitaminosis D may lead to nephritis and other degenerative renal changes [21]. Profound vitamin A deficiency causes squamous metaplasia of ureteral mucosa and collecting ducts leading to blockage of the ureters and secondary hydronephrosis, hyperuricemia, and oliguric/anuric renal failure [2,4].

Excess vitamin D_3 promotes metastatic mineralization of viscera including the kidney [15,22,23]. This problem most commonly affects nestling parrots [15]. Clinical signs may include polyuria/polydipsia, anorexia, crop stasis, and weight loss [14,22]. The recommended level of vitamin D_3 for chickens is 300 IU/kg feed. Toxic effects reportedly occur with vitamin D_3 levels exceeding 1000 IU/kg feed [23].

Inflammatory causes of renal disease

Renal amyloidosis is most common in captive, adult waterfowl, shore-birds, cranes, flamingos, and songbirds [4,15,24]. Amyloidosis is often associated with chronic inflammatory conditions such as sepsis, gout, enteritis, and arthritis [24–26].

Infectious causes of renal disease

The absence of lymph nodes and the presence of renal and hepatic portal systems increase the risk of systemic or gastrointestinal microbes affecting the kidney [27,28].

Viral nephritis

Avian polyomavirus is the most important cause of viral nephritis in the companion psittacine bird. Up to 70% of affected non-budgerigar psittacines develop glomerulopathy characterized by immune complex deposition, but affected birds die acutely from other problems without showing signs of renal disease [4,15,26,29–31].

Other viruses with tropism for the avian kidney include infectious bronchitis virus, picornavirus, paramyxoviruses such as Newcastle disease virus, influenza virus, and togaviruses [12,15,27,32–34]. Infectious bronchitis virus is an important cause of renal disease and urolithiasis in galliforms [12,15,32]. Lymphoplasmacytic interstitial nephritis is common in birds infected with West Nile virus but only as a part of generalized disease [15,35].

Bacterial nephritis

Bacterial nephritis usually occurs when bacteria enter the kidney secondary to systemic disease through the renal arteries or the renal portal system [4,26]. Rarely, bacteria ascend the ureters secondary to conditions such as chronic cloacitis [4,23,26]. A wide range of bacteria has been reported to cause bacterial nephritis including Enterobacteriaceae, *Pasteurella* spp, *Pseudomonas* spp, *Streptococcus* spp, and *Staphylococcus* spp [4,15,26,27]. *Listeria monocytogenes* has been reported in raptors [15,26], whereas *Erysipelothrix rhusiopathiae* has been reported in quail and chicken [15,26,36]. *Mycobacterium avium* can, rarely, cause renal lesions [15,37].

Chlamydial nephritis

Chlamydial nephritis is poorly documented [4,38]. In a survey of 23 birds with psittacosis, 35% had renal congestion, bile pigment nephrosis, and glomerulopathy, but *Chlamydophila psittaci* could not be detected in renal tissue [26]. Identification of chlamydial organisms in the avian kidney has been reported in only two juvenile parrots [38].

Fungal nephritis

Fungi are a rare cause of renal disease [4,39]. Lesions may develop from fungal invasion of vessels or extension from air sacs [15].

Parasitic nephritis

Renal coccidiosis is the most important cause of parasitic nephritis. Disease caused by the coccidian *Eimeria* spp is most common in free-ranging, juvenile waterfowl [40,41]. Disease has also been described in the domestic goose (*Anser anser domesticus*) and aquatic birds such as the loon (*Gavia immer*), gull (*Larus argentatus*), puffin (*Fratercula arctica*), cormorant (*Phalacrocorax auritus*), woodcock (*Scolopax minor*), and penguin (*Eudyptula minor*) [14,15,42–45]. Renal coccidiosis is less commonly reported in raptors [15]. Although renal coccidiosis is often asymptomatic, emaciation, acute renal failure, and death may occur secondary to granulomatous interstitial nephritis [14,46,47].

The microsporidian, *Encephalitozoon hellem*, may also cause severe granulomatous nephritis [14,26,46,48–50], although the presence of microsporidians in the kidney or urine can be incidental [14,15,51]. Renal microsporidiosis is most commonly reported in the lovebird (*Agapornis* spp), particularly those positive for psittacine beak and feather disease [50,51]. There are also reports of renal microsporidiosis in the budgerigar, eclectus (Eclectus roratus), and red-bellied parrot (*Poicephalus rufiventris*) [51,52].

Traumatic causes of avian renal disease

In mammals, crush injuries and other conditions causing muscle necrosis are known to cause tubular changes, myoglobin cast formation, and renal failure, [14] Myogobinuria has been reported in flamingo (*Phoenicopterus* sp) and ostrich (*Struthio camelus*) with capture myopathy, and there is one report of renal failure in an ostrich with extensive muscle necrosis and marked hyperuricemia [14,27].

Direct trauma is rare because the avian kidneys are so well protected by bone [7]. If a renal hematoma does develop, it can apply pressure to spinal nerves causing limb paresis [27]. Crushing of the kidney may also occur during dystocia [46].

Toxic nephropathies in the avian patient

Because of the presence of renal and hepatic portal systems, the avian kidney is frequently affected by toxins in the avian gut such as heavy metals, anti-inflammatory agents, and antibiotics [28]. Lead toxicity is associated with acute tubular necrosis or nephrosis and visceral gout [53].

The nonsteroidal anti-inflammatory agent flunixin has been implicated in presumptive nephrotoxicity of cranes and flamingos [54]. In northern bobwhite quail (*Colinus virginianus*), doses of flunixin as low as 0.1 mg/kg led to the development of gout [54]. Another nonsteroidal anti-inflammatory agent, diclofenac, has been linked to renal failure, visceral gout, and high death rates in vultures of the Indian subcontinent [55].

Most information regarding antibiotic nephrotoxicity is based on studies in mammals. For instance, renal tubules accumulate aminoglycoside potentially leading to nephrotoxicity in mammals [56]. Gentamicin may be more likely to cause nephrotoxicity in the bird because polyuria/polydipsia is often seen even at low doses [56]. Gentamicin (5 mg/kg intramuscularly every 12 hours for 7 days) led to profound polyuria/polydipsia in cockatoos (*Eolophus sp*) which persisted for 23 days after stopping treatment [57]. Loss of balance, impaired vision, and muscle spasms were described in two falcons (*Falco biarmicus*) given gentamicin (5 mg/kg/d for 4 days) [58]. Amikacin is considered the least nephrotoxic of the aminoglycosides, but transient polyuria/polydipsia may still occur [59].

A host of other drugs and toxins have been associated with renal lesions in birds, including dexamethasone, medroxyprogesterone, aflatoxins, mycotoxins, herbicides, and vitamin D_3-based rodenticides [15,46,60,61]. There are also reports of oak toxicity in a cassowary (*Casuarius casuarius*) [62] and of ethylene glycol poisoning in geese [63].

Postrenal disease

Conditions such as urolithiasis, dystocia, cloacal, or coelomic masses and, in rare instances, ureteral tumors may cause mechanical compression or obstruction of the avian ureter [7,64].

Urolithiasis and visceral gout

Urolithiasis and visceral gout are important causes of renal failure in pullets and caged laying hens. These conditions are seen only sporadically in companion birds [2,28]. Visceral gout is defined as the accumulation of uric acid tophi on serosal surfaces of the pericardium, liver capsule, air sacs, and within the kidney but may be found any tissue [26]. Urolithiasis is simply the presence of urinary tract calculi.

The pathogenesis of gout is not completely understood, but gout is generally associated with conditions that reduce uric acid excretion or increase uric acid production [2,23,65]:

Reduced uric acid excretion Increased uric acid production
Dehydration
Excess dietary calcium
Renal tubular disease
Excess dietary protein

Infectious renal disease
Hypovitaminosis A
Obstructive ureteral disease

Urolith development is most commonly associated with severe dehydration; other factors may include excess dietary calcium, dietary electrolyte imbalances, infectious bronchitis virus, *Mycoplasma synoviae* infection, mycotoxicosis, or shipping stress [12,13,66–68]. Excess dietary protein has also been correlated with increased production of uric acid, but even with very high levels of dietary protein (ie, 80%) gout develops only in genetically susceptible individuals [69,70]. Nevertheless, it is still theorized that long-term of high-protein feeding may induce hyperuricemia in granivorous or nectivorous birds [23,71].

The presence of uroliths in the kidney leads to compensatory hypertrophy of remaining renal tissue. Affected birds often appear normal until ureteral flow from the contralateral kidney is blocked, leading to lethargy, straining, and death [27,66,67]. Visceral gout is rarely diagnosed ante mortem, and birds are usually found dead [4].

Articular gout

Articular gout is defined as the accumulation of uric acid tophi in or around joints. Articular gout lesions are particularly common on the foot and hock [65]. Clinical signs of articular gout may include reluctance to move, shifting from leg to leg, lameness, and joint swelling [4].

Diagnosis

Early recognition and diagnosis of renal disease is extremely challenging, but an early definitive diagnosis provides the best opportunity for helping the patient [3].

Clinical pathology

In advanced renal disease, normocytic-normochromic anemia, hyperuricemia, uremia, and changes in plasma electrolyte, calcium, and phosphorus levels may be detected [72]. Uric acid excretion is largely independent of urine flow and therefore is unaffected by moderate changes in glomerular filtration [72]. Elevations in uric acid (up to 20 mg/dL) may be seen with severe dehydration [23,73,74], but uric acid does not increase significantly with renal disease unless there is extensive tubular damage [75]. Postprandial hyperuricemia may occur for up to 8 hours in carnivorous birds [76,77].

Urea nitrogen (BUN) has little value in the detection of renal disease in most birds [4,73], but BUN is a sensitive indicator of hydration. In the dehydrated bird, up to 99% of BUN is reabsorbed. A significant postprandial elevation in BUN has also been documented in healthy raptors [77].

The avian kidney cannot concentrate sodium or electrolytes much above normal levels [78]. Possible findings with renal failure may include hyponatremia, hyperkalemia, hypocalcemia, and hyperphosphatemia [27], although elevations in phosphorus are not commonly recognized in avian renal disease [72,74]. Alterations in these electrolytes have been inconsistently reported in active cases of avian renal disease. No definitive correlations between electrolyte abnormalities and renal disease in birds have been made.

Urinalysis

Urine flows from the ureters into the urodeum and then enters the colon and, in some species, the cecum or ileum, by reverse peristalsis (Fig. 1) [79,80]. Columnar epithelial cells lining the urodeum and colon modify ureteral urine through the absorption or secretion of water, electrolytes, and nitrogen [78]. Important indications for urinalysis include persistent biochemical or radiographic abnormalities consistent with renal disease or persistent polyuria (Fig. 2) [14]. Causes of polyuria are extensive and nonspecific and include fluid therapy, renal disease, liver disease, gastrointestinal disease, diabetes mellitus, and pituitary tumors [4,14]. Polyuria may also occur with sepsis even when the pathogen does not directly affect the kidney, and psychogenic polydipsia has been reported in one African gray parrot (*Psittacus erithacus*) [14,81]. A common cause of polyuria and pollakiuria in the avian patient is stress [14,82].

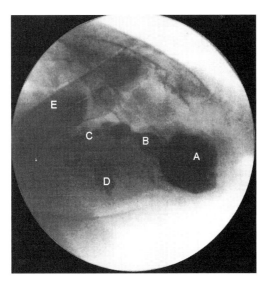

Fig. 1. Retroperistalsis of urereteral urine from cloaca (*A*) into avian large intestine (*B, C, D*). (*E*) the femurs. (*From* Brummermann M, Braun EJ. Effect of salt and water balance on colonic motility of white leghorn roosters. Am J Physiol Regulatory Integrative Comp Physiol 1995;268:690–8; with permission.)

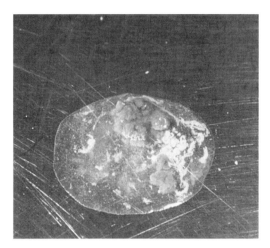

Fig. 2. Polyuria in a bird dropping. Notice the large ring of urine around the feces and urates. (*Courtesy of* Ed Ramsay, DVM, DACZM.)

Although cloacal cannulation techniques have been described [83], free-catch urine samples are always collected from clinical patients. Obtain fresh urine samples free of urates and feces from clean, nonabsorbent surfaces such as wax paper [3,14,23,46]. A free-catch urine sample does not necessarily represent ureteral urine, and this fact should be taken into account when interpreting the results.

Birds possess a limited ability to concentrate urine, making avian urine isosmotic or slightly hyperosmotic. Urine specific gravity normally ranges from 1.005 to 1.020 g/mL but is highly variable among the different species. Urine specific gravity is not particularly useful unless values are consistently low [14,46].

Urine color

Pigments present in feces or newspaper can leach into urine and urates over time [14,23]. In the anorectic bird, concentrated bile pigments create emerald green or black feces that may stain urine even before droppings are passed [23]. Liver dysfunction or, in rare instances, hemolysis, may lead to biliverdinuria or lime-green, yellow, or, less commonly, orange urine and urates [14,23,46].

Red urine may be seen with hematuria, hemoglobinuria, or myoglobinuria. Hemoglobinuria may be seen in Amazon parrots (*Amazona* spp) with lead toxicosis producing dark red, pink, or tan/brown urates [4,23]. Hematuria may be associated with renal neoplasia, nephritis, or toxic nephropathy, although blood can also originate from the intestinal or reproductive tracts [4,23]. Transient wine-colored urine may occur in chicks, especially African gray and eclectus parrots. This condition may be correlated with hand-feeding animal protein–based diets [4,14,23].

Urine dipstick parameters

The pH of avian urine typically ranges from 6.0 to 8.0 [14,46,9]. Urine pH may be influenced by diet and cloacal contents [23,46], with urine more acidic in laying hens and more alkaline with bacterial metabolism [84]. Glucose levels in urine are normally zero to trace, although biliverdinuria may interfere with urine protein readings [23,46]. Normal avian urine is also free of ketones except during starvation or migration, when metabolism switches to beta-oxidation of fats [23,26]. Standard mammalian urine dipstick tests should be interpreted with caution, because these tests are not designed or calibrated for accuracy with avian species.

Urine sediment

Lane [46] recommends centrifugation of urine for 1 to 2 minutes. Normal sediment contains many squamous epithelial cells and amorphous urate, calcium oxalate, and sulfonamide crystals [46]. Low numbers of red and white cells (<3/high power field, $\times$ 40) are present in avian urine. There should also be small numbers of bacteria present that are probably from fecal or cloacal contamination [14,23,46]. Normal bird urine contains no casts. Granular, hemoglobin, and other casts are reported in the literature and may be associated with renal disease [14,46].

Blood culture

To identify the cause of sepsis and bacterial nephritis, blood culture is a much better test than urine culture [14].

Radiographs

The avian kidney is difficult to evaluate radiographically because of its position within the synsacral fossa. Obscured by parenchyma on the ventrodorsal view, the kidneys are best viewed on the lateral projection. The most consistent radiographic sign of renomegaly is enlargement of the cranial renal division, which is best appreciated on the lateral view. Enlargement of this cranial renal division will also make the kidneys more apparent on the ventrodorsal view [3,7]. Renomegaly will also cause the wedge of air sac space separating the kidneys and coelomic viscera to become diminished in the lateral view. There may also be loss of the air sac diverticulum separating the dorsal renal surface from the ventral synsacrum [23]. Marked renomegaly may displace the ventriculus ventrally or caudoventrally [4]. Positive contrast radiography may make evaluation of the kidneys easier by helping outline coelomic structures [4,28]. Intravenous excretory urography may also provide more information on renal size, shape, and function [27,28].

Increased renal opacity may be associated with small kidney size, dehydration, or renal mineralization (Fig. 3) [3,4,23]. Urate tophi are not

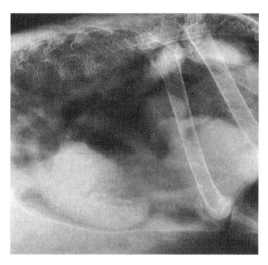

Fig. 3. Radiopacity of kidneys in a spectacled owl (*Pulsatrix perspicillata*) on the lateral view.

normally evident radiographically, but congestion of urates secondary to obstruction or gout may also lead to opacification [7]. Although the normal avian kidneys are more difficult to evaluate on the ventrodorsal view, they will become prominent with radiopacity (Fig. 4) [7,27].

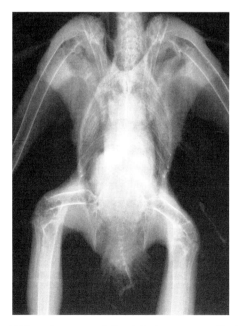

Fig. 4. Radiopacity of kidneys in a spectacled owl (*Pulsatrix perspicillata*) on the ventrodorsal projection.

Ultrasonography

Because of the dorsal position of the avian kidney and the presence of air sacs, ultrasound is generally impossible in the normal bird [5,85]. Transcloacal ultrasound of the normal kidney has been described in large birds [86]. In smaller birds, organomegaly or ascites may compress the abdominal air sacs enough to create an acoustic window [5,23,85].

Alternate imaging

CT or MRI may prove helpful for evaluation of the renal system [87].

Laparoscopy

Laparoscopic renal biopsy is the best ante mortem diagnostic test for avian renal disease [4]. Indications for renal biopsy include persistent polyuria/polydipsia and serum biochemical abnormalities, gout, radiographic abnormalities of the kidneys, or abnormal urinalysis results, particularly the presence of casts [1,4,8]. Renal biopsy should be avoided in patients with a single kidney, cystic kidneys, renal abscesses, or hydronephrosis [1,3].

The standard entry site for laparoscopy is the caudal thoracic air sac [3,28]. A caudal entry site dorsal to the pubis and caudal to the ischium allows better access and visualization of the caudal renal division, but this site should be avoided in raptors because the presence of large tail muscles increases the risk of hemorrhage [28].

There are conflicting recommendations on where to biopsy the avian kidney. Muller [1] has recommended the cranial renal division because of its size and visibility, but the middle or caudal divisions may be safer sites. The cranial renal artery reportedly lies more superficial and therefore is more easily lacerated or torn during biopsy [28,88].

Diagnosis of gout

Cytologic evaluation of gouty lesions reveals uric acid crystals and inflammatory cells. The murexide test can be used to confirm the presence of urates. Nitric acid is mixed with crystals on a slide that is slowly flame dried. If red or purple color appears after ammonia is added, urates are present [4]. Histologically, urates are demonstrated by using alcohol fixation and special stains [28].

Renal scintigraphy

Given the challenges of obtaining a nonmodified ureteral urine sample, scintigraphy is a potentially useful method to evaluate renal function [89]. Methods have been described in the chicken, pigeon, and cockatiel (*Nymphicus hollandicus*) [7,89,90].

Systemic arterial blood pressure

Currently, blood pressure is not easily or routinely measured in the bird. In chickens, glomerular filtration is maintained over pressures ranging from 40 to 110 mm Hg [91].

Therapeutics

Management of renal failure should focus on delaying or halting progression of disease and treatment of sequelae. If the cause of the renal failure is known, specific therapy should be instituted. Although severe loss of renal tissue is permanently disabling, survival for extended periods is possible with only a small proportion of normal renal tissue.

Supportive care

Treat dehydration rapidly to prevent exacerbation of renal disease [28]. In renal failure, provide aggressive fluid therapy. Maintenance fluid requirements are estimated as 40 to 50 mL/kg/d in many species. Providing twice the required maintenance volume of fluids is a good initial goal for many patients. Replace only insensible fluid loss in anuric or oliguric birds (20–25 mL/kg/d) [28,78]. Weigh all birds receiving fluids twice daily.

Provide nutrition high in fat and carbohydrates and low in protein, potassium, phosphorus, and sodium in mild to moderate renal failure in granivorous and nectivorous species [4,28]. Products such as psittacine hand-feeding formula and low-protein products have been recommended [4,28]. Dietary restriction of protein may relieve some clinical signs of renal failure such as nausea. A diet restricted in protein and minerals also reduces the serum phosphorus levels, which may slow the progression of renal disease. Never the less, low-protein diets may lead to malnutrition, and low-protein diets are contraindicated in patients with advanced renal failure [92].

In the dog, research has suggested that omega-3 polyunsaturated fatty acid (PUFA) supplementation may preserve renal function and delay the progression of renal disease [93]. Omega-3 PUFA are abundant in fish oil [93,94]. Although the precise mechanism is not fully understood [93], omega-3 PUFA may work particularly well in animal models of renal disease that involve an immune component [94], a form of renal disease which is rare in the avian patient [15]. Administer omega-3 fatty acids for 6 to 12 months (S. Echols, personal communication, 2005).

Medical management

Drugs used to treat avian renal disease are listed in Table 1.

If dietary restriction of protein is unsuccessful in maintaining a normal level of serum phosphorus, hyperphosphatemia may be managed with oral phosphate binders. Hypocalcemia may require calcium supplementation. Depending on the underlying cause of disease, other drugs that may be indicated include anti-inflammatory agents in amyloidosis and parenteral vitamin A in individuals with a deficient diet [4,8,28].

Volume overload is best prevented rather than treated, but diuretics such as furosemide or mannitol or renal vasodilators such as dopamine may be indicated if the animal is well hydrated and urine production is poor [4,92,96]. In confirmed or suspected cases of bacterial nephritis, choose antibiotics that achieve adequate renal tissue levels such as fluoroquinolones [28,56,97]. Antibiotics should also ideally be bactericidal. Cephalosporins are considered an excellent choice for urinary tract disease in the mammal, but the degree of biotransformation and routes of excretion are unknown in the bird [97]. Avoid nephrotoxic medications such as aminoglycoside antibiotics and other potential renal toxins (Box 1). Sulfa drugs should be avoided in dehydrated patients because sulfonamides possess a low water solubility and may precipitate in mammalian kidneys [56]. Differences in the organization of collecting ducts and ureteral branching in the bird may predispose certain avian species to obstructive nephropathies resulting from drug precipitation [56]. Administer antibiotics for at least 4 to 6 weeks (S. Echols, personal communication).

Hyperuricemia may respond to allopurinol or colchicine, although allopurinol can induce hyperuricemia and gout in the red-tailed hawk (*Buteo jamaicensis*) [95]. The recombinant enzyme, urate oxidase, shows great potential for the treatment of hyperuricemia in pigeons and red-tailed hawks [98]. Continue therapy with colchicine or allopurinol until signs of gout are gone and the patient is well stabilized (S. Echols, personal communication).

Administration of a histamine-receptor antagonist such as cimetidine or famotidine decreases gastric acidity and vomiting. Multiple B-vitamin preparations should be given to compensate for urinary losses of water-soluble vitamins [92].

Treatment for anemia may include iron supplementation and anabolic steroids such as nandrolone to stimulate erythrocyte production. Recombinant erythropoietin may also be effective in stimulating red blood cell production in birds showing clinical signs of anemia. Anti-erythropoietin antibodies are known to develop in a significant percentage of mammals, leading to refractory anemia [92].

In mammals, peritoneal dialysis or hemodialysis is ideally initiated when signs of renal disease are present and are not treatable by other forms of medical management. The use of dialysis has not been described in the avian patient.

Management of renal tumors

Nephrectomy is the treatment of choice for unilateral renal tumors in the dog [92]. Unfortunately, renal tumors are exceedingly difficult to manage

Table 1
Drugs used in avian renal disease

Drug	Dosage	Indications	Comments
Allopurinol	10–15 mg/kg PO q 12 h	Hyperuricemia	Do not give to red-tailed hawks and possibly other birds of prey; maintain hydration; use with amoxicillin/clavulanate or aspirin is contraindicated
Aluminum hydroxide	30–90 mg/kg PO q 12 h	Phosphate binder	Compounds containing aluminum may interfere with fluoroquinolone absorption
Amoxicillin	20–100 mg/kg PO q 12–24 h	Bacterial nephritis	
Amoxicillin/clavulanate	125 mg/kg PO q 8 h	Bacterial nephritis	Use with allopurinol is contraindicated
Butorphanol	0.5–4.0 mg/kg IM q 4–6 h	Analgesia, renal tumors	
Calcium glubionate	25–150 mg/kg PO q 12–24 h	Hypocalcemia, hyperphosphatemia	If the calcium × phosphorus (Ca × P) product exceeds 70, metastatic mineralization is likely to occur as in mammals; compounds containing calcium may interfere with tetracycline and fluoroquinolone absorption
Calcium gluconate (10%)	25–100 mg/kg SC, IM q 12 h	Hypocalcemia, hyperphosphatemia	Dilute 1:1 with sterile water, saline; compounds containing calcium may interfere with tetracycline and fluoroquinolone absorption
Cefotaxime	75–100 mg/kg IM, IV q 4–8 h	Bacterial nephritis	
Cefoxitin	50–100 mg/kg IM, IV q 6–12 h	Bacterial nephritis	
Ceftazidime	50–100 mg/kg IM, IV q 4–8 h	Bacterial nephritis	
Ceftiofur	10 mg/kg IM q 4–12 h 50–100 mg/kg IM q 4–8 h	Bacterial nephritis	Administration q 4 h recommended in cockatiels based on pharmacokinetic data
Ceftriaxone	100 mg/kg IM q 4 h	Bacterial nephritis	
Cimetidine	5 mg/kg PO, IM q 8–12 h	Nausea	
Ciprofloxacin	50 mg/kg PO, IV 12h	Bacterial nephritis	
Colchicine	0.01–0.04 mg/kg PO q 12–24 h	Hyperuricemia	Gradually increase dose to q 12 h; may exacerbate gout in some cases

Drug	Dosage	Indication	Comments
Enrofloxacin	10–15 mg/kg PO, SC, IM q 12 h	Bacterial nephritis	Compounds containing calcium, aluminum interfere with absorption
Furosemide	0.1–2.0 mg/kg PO, SC, IM, IV q 6–12 h; 1–4 mg/kg PO, SC, IM. IV q 6–12 h	Volume overload	Lower dosage range recommended for raptors and nectivorous birds
Iron dextran	10 mg/kg IM, repeat in 7–10 d	Anemia	Use cautiously in species in which iron storage disease is common (toucans, mynahs)
Mannitol	0.25–2.0 mg/kg q 24 h IV (slow bolus)	Volume overload	Osmotic diuretic
Meloxicam	0.5 mg/kg q 1 h PO, SC	Analgesia in the palliative treatment of renal tumors; amyloidosis	Potentially the least nephrotoxic of the nonsteroidal agents
Metoclopramide	0.5 mg/kg PO, IM, IV q 8 h	Gastrointestinal ileus; crop stasis	
Methylprednisolone acetate	0.5–1.0 mg/kg PO, IM	Renal tumor, palliative	
Nandrolone laurate	0.2–2.0 mg/kg SC, IM once or q 3 wk	Anemia; chronic renal failure	
Norfloxacin	8–10 mg/kg PO q 24 h	Bacterial nephritis	
Omega-3 fatty acids	0.1–0.2 mL/kg flaxseed oil: corn oil mixed at a ratio of 1:4 PO SID or added to food	Glomerulopathy	Consider vitamin E supplementation with long-term use
Potassium chloride	20–40 mEq/L fluids	Diuresis, hypokalemia	
Urate oxidase	100–200 IU/kg IM q 24 h	Hyperuricemia	Currently very expensive
Vitamin A	2000–5000 IU/kg IM once or q 24 h × 14 d, followed by 250–1000 IU/kg q 24 h PO	Hypovitaminosis A	Chronic use may lead to vitamin A toxicity.
Vitamin B complex	1–2 mL/L fluids	Renal failure, supportive care	

Data from Pollock CG, Carpenter JW, Antinoff N. Birds. In: Carpenter JW, editor. Exotic animal formulary. 3rd edition. St. Louis (MO): Elsevier Saunders; 2005. p. 135–344; Lumeij JT, Redig PT. Hyperuricemia and visceral gout induced by allopurinol in red-tailed hawks (*Buteo jamaicensis*). In: Proceedings Tagung der Fachgruppe Gefluegelkrankheiten, Giessen, Germany: Deutsche Veterinaermedizinische Gesellschaft; 1992.

Box 1. Drugs with known potential for nephrotoxicity[a]

Aminoglycosides particularly gentamicin
Amphotericin B[b]
Calcium EDTA
Chloramphenicol
Cisplatin
Deferoxamine
Enalapril
Flunixin meglumine and other non-steroidal anti-inflammatory
   agents
Nystatin[c]
Paramomycin[d]
Polymyxin B
Sulfanomides[e]
Tetracyclines[f]

---

[a] If potentially nephrotoxic agents must be used, monitor patients closely for clinical signs of nephrotoxicity such as polyuria/polydipsia, monitor serum/plasma uric acid levels and maintain hydration. Most knowledge regarding nephrotoxicity is based upon information gained from mammals; the drugs listed are not the only potentially nephrotoxic agents available.

[b] Amphotericin B is highly nephrotoxic in mammals, however nephrotoxicity has not been documented in birds with even long-term treatment.

[c] Nephrotoxicity may occur if nystatin is systemically absorbed due to the presence of erosions and ulcers lining the gastrointestinal tract.

[d] Nephrotoxicity may occur if ulcerative bowel lesions are present and systemic absorption occurs.

[e] Sulfa drugs are known to possess low water solubility, and may precipitate in renal tubules in the face of dehydration.

[f] High doses of tetracycline or outdated tetracycline may cause acute tubular nephrosis.

Data from Refs. [1,56,59].

---

surgically in the bird because of the kidney's dorsal location, the vascular nature of these tumors, and the likelihood of regional invasion into nearby tissues [4,10].

Palliative treatment is more commonly chosen for management of renal tumors and may include analgesics and steroids such as methylprednisolone [4,99]. In mammals, chemotherapy has not been shown to be effective against renal tumors other than lymphosarcoma [92], and the use of chemotherapy has been little evaluated for avian renal tumors. Use of carboplatin (5 mg/kg intravenously) in a parakeet dramatically improved limb use, although the mass continued to enlarge [100].

Treatment of urolithiasis

Treatment of urolithiasis is generally not attempted in domestic fowl, the type of bird most frequently affected by this condition. The primary goal in the treatment of obstructive uropathy is to relieve blockage of urine flow. There is one description of surgical removal of ureteroliths in a companion parrot and one report on the use of lithotripsy for urolithiasis in a Magellanic penguin (*Spheniscus magellanicus*) [64,101].

Fluid therapy, ideally administered by an intravenous or intraosseous route, improves renal function and corrects electrolyte abnormalities after the obstruction has been relieved. Normal saline is the fluid of choice. Large quantities of fluids may be required because postobstructive diuresis may occur for 1 to 5 days. Carefully monitor urine output, body weight, serum electrolytes, hematocrit, and total protein levels [92].

Summary

Renal disease in the avian patient is probably under-recognized. An important reason may be the subtle nature of clinical signs until disease is quite advanced. Common diagnostic tests performed in the diagnosis of renal disease include a complete blood cell count, chemistry panel, urinalysis, survey radiographs, and laparoscopic evaluation and biopsy of the kidneys. Depending on the patient's signs, history, and physical examination findings, additional diagnostic tests may include heavy metal blood levels, fecal flotation, blood culture, and viral serologic tests. Important underlying causes of renal disease in the avian patient include renal coccidiosis in waterfowl, dehydration, toxicosis, systemic bacterial infection, and amyloidosis. Primary renal tumors are relatively uncommon in birds with the notable exception of the budgerigar parakeet. When gout is present, it should generally be considered as a clinical manifestation of severe renal dysfunction [4,78]. The mainstay of treatment for renal disease in the bird is supportive care such as fluid therapy and nutritional support. Additional therapy should ideally be tailored to the underlying pathogenesis of disease and specific sequelae.

References

[1] Muller K, Gobel T, Muller S, et al. Use of endoscopy and renal biopsy for the diagnosis of kidney disease in free-living birds of prey and owls. Vet Rec 2004;155(11):326–9.

[2] Siller WG. Renal pathology of the fowl- a review. Avian Pathol 1981;10:187–262.

[3] Murray MJ, Taylor M. Avian renal disease: endoscopic applications. Seminars in Avian and Exotic Pet Medicine 1999;8(3):115–21.

[4] Speer BL. Diseases of the urogenital system. In: Altman RB, Clubb SL, Dorrestein GM, et al, editors. Avian medicine and surgery. Philadelphia: WB Saunders; 1997. p. 625–44.

[5] Canny C. Gross anatomy and imaging of the avian and reptilian urinary system. Seminars in Avian and Exotic Pet Medicine 1998;7(2):72–80.

[6] Gevaert D, Nelis J, Verhaeghe B. Plasma chemistry and urine analysis in Salmonella-induced polyuria in racing pigeons (*Columbia livia*). Avian Pathol 1991;20:379–86.

[7] McMillan MC. Imaging of avian urogenital disorders. AAV Today 1988;2(2):74–82.

[8] Echols MS. Antemortem diagnosis and management of avian renal disease. In: Association of Avian Veterinarians Annual Conference Proceedings. St. Paul (MN): 1998. p. 83–90.

[9] Van Toor AJ, Zwart P, et al. Adenocarcinoma of the kidney in two budgerigars. Avian Pathol 1984;13:145–50.

[10] Freeman KP, Hahn KA, Jones MP, et al. Right leg muscle atrophy and osteopenia caused by renal adenocarcinoma in a cockatiel (*Melopsittacus undulatus*). Vet Radiol Ultrasound 1999;40(2):144–7.

[11] Neuman U, Kummerfeld N. Neoplasms in budgerigars (*Melopsittacus undulatus*): clinical, pathomorphological and serological findings with special consideration of kidney tumours. Avian Pathol 1983;12:353–62.

[12] Cowen BS, Wideman RF, Rothenbacher H. An outbreak of avian urolithiasis on a large commercial egg farm. Avian Dis 1987;31:392–7.

[13] Julian R. Water deprivation as a cause of renal disease of chickens. Avian Pathol 1982;11:615–7.

[14] Phalen D. Avian renal disorders. In: Fudge AM, editor. Laboratory medicine avian and exotic pets. Philadelphia: WB Saunders; 2000. p. 61–8.

[15] Schmidt RE, Reavill DR, Phalen DN. Urinary system. In: Pathology of pet and aviary birds. Ames (IA): Iowa State Press; 2003. p. 95–107.

[16] Forbes NA, Cooper JE. Fatty liver-kidney syndrome of merlins. In: Redig PT, Cooper JE, Remple D, et al, editors. Raptor biomedicine. Minneapolis (MN): University of Minnesota Press; 1993. p. 45–8.

[17] Pearce J, Balnave D. A review of biotin deficiency and fatty liver and kidney syndrome in poultry. Br Vet J 1978;134(6):598–608.

[18] Howerth EW, Schorr LF, Nettles VF. Neoplasia in free-flying ruffed grouse (*Bonasa umbellus*). Avian Dis 1986;30(1):238–40.

[19] Hubbard GB. Renal carcinoma in a captive Edwards lorry (*Trichoglossus haematodus capistratus*). J Wildl Dis 1983;19(2):160–1.

[20] Latimer KS, Ritchie BW, Campagnoli RP, et al. Metastatic renal carcinoma in an African grey parrot (*Psittacus erithacus erithacus*). J Vet Diagn Invest 1996;8:261–4.

[21] Chandra M, Singh B, Soni GL, et al. Renal and biochemical changes produced in broilers by high-protein, high-calcium, urea-containing, and vitamin-A-deficient diets. Avian Dis 1984;8(1):1–11.

[22] Schoemaker NJ, Lumeij JT, Beynen AC. Polyuria and polydipsia due to vitamin and mineral oversupplementation of the diet of a salmon crested cockatoo (Cacatua moluccensis) and blue and gold macaw (*Ara ararauna*). Avian Pathol 1997;26:201–9.

[23] Styles DK, Phalen DN. Clinical avian urology. Seminars in Avian and Exotic Pet Medicine 1998;7(2):104–13.

[24] Schneider RR, Hunter DB, Waltner-Toews D, et al. A descriptive study of mortality at the Kortright waterfowl park 1982–1986. Can Vet J 1988;29:911–4.

[25] Nakamura K, Tanaka H, Kodama Y, et al. Systemic amyloidosis in laying Japanese quail. Avian Dis 1998;42(1):209–14.

[26] Phalen DN, Ambrus S, Graham DL. The avian urinary system: form, function, diseases. In: Association of Avian Veterinarians Annual Conference Proceedings. Boca Raton (FL): Association of Avian Veterinarians; 1990. p. 44–57.

[27] Lierz M. Avian renal disease: pathogenesis, diagnosis, and therapy. Vet Clin North Am Exotic Am Pract 2003;6:29–55.

[28] Lumeij JT. Pathophysiology, diagnosis and treatment of renal disorders in birds of prey. In: Lumeij JT, Remple D, Redig PT, et al, editors. Raptor biomedicine III. Lake Worth (FL): Zoological Education Network, Inc; 2000. p. 169–78.

[29] Gerlach H, Enders F, Casares M, et al. Membranous glomerulopathy as an indicator of avian polyomavirus infection in Psittaciformes. J Avian Med Surg 1998;12(4): 248–54.

[30] Lafferty SL, Fudge AM, Schmidt RE, et al. Avian polyomavirus infection and disease in a green aracaris (*Pteroglossus viridis*). Avian Dis 1999;43(3):577–85.

[31] Phalen DN, Wilson VG, Graham DL. Characterization of the avian polyomavirus-associated glomerulopathy of nestling parrots. Avian Dis 1996;40(1):140–9.

[32] Lee CW, Brown C, Hilt DA, et al. Nephropathogenesis of chickens experimentally infected with various strains of infectious bronchitis virus. J Vet Med Sci 2004;66(7): 835–40.

[33] Swayne DE, Radin MJ, Hoepf TM, et al. Acute renal failure as the cause of death in chickens following intravenous inoculation with avian influenza virus A/chicken/Alabama/7395/ 75 (H4N8). Avian Dis 1994;38(1):151–7.

[34] Ziegler AF, Ladman BS, Dunn PA, et al. Nephropathogenic infectious bronchitis in Pennsylvania chickens 1997–2000. Avian Dis 2002;46(4):847–58.

[35] Kramer LD, Bernard KA. West Nile virus infection in birds and mammals. Ann N Y Acad Sci 2001;951:84–93.

[36] Mutalib A, Keirs R, Austin F. Erysipelas in quail and suspected erysipeloid in processing plant employees. Avian Dis 1995;39(1):191–3.

[37] Sato Y, Aoyagi T, Matsuura S, et al. An occurrence of avian tuberculosis in hooded merganser (*Lophodytes cucullatus*). Avian Dis 1996;40(4):941–4.

[38] Shivaprasad HL, Crespo R, Woolcock PR, et al. Unusual cases of Chlamydiosis in psittacines. In: Association of Avian Veterinarians Annual Conference Proceedings. Monterey (CA): 2002, p. 205–7.

[39] Tham VL, Purcell DA, Schultz DJ. Fungal nephritis in a grey-headed albatross. J Wildl Dis 1974;10:306–9.

[40] Gajadhar AA, Cawthorn RJ, Wobeser GA, et al. Prevalence of renal coccidia in wild waterfowl in Saskatchewan. Can J Zool 1983;61:2631–3.

[41] Leighton FA, Gajadhar AA. *Eimeria fraterculae* sp. n. in the kidneys of Atlantic puffins (*Fratercula arctica*) from Newfoundland, Canada: species description and lesions. J Wildl Dis 1986;22(4):520–6.

[42] Gajadhar AA, Leighton FA. *Eimeria wobeseri* sp. n. and *Eimeria goelandi* sp. n. (Protozoa: Apicomplexa) in the kidneys of herring gulls (*Larus argentatus*). J Wildl Dis 1988;24(3): 538–46.

[43] Montgomery RD, Novilla MN, Shillinger RB. Renal coccidiosis caused by *Eimeria gavia* n. sp. in a common loon (*Gavia immer*). Avian Dis 1978;22(4):809–14.

[44] Obendorf DL, McColl K. Mortality in little penguins (*Eudyptula minor*) along the coast of Victoria, Australia. J Wildl Dis 1989;16(2):251–9.

[45] Yabsley MJ, Gottdenker NL, Fischer JR. Description of a new *Eimeria* sp. and associated lesions in the kidneys of double-crested cormorants (*Phalocrocorax auritus*). J Parasitol 2002;88(6):1230–3.

[46] Lane RA. Avian urinalysis a practical guide to analysis and interpretation. In: Rosskopf WJ, Woerpel RW, editors. Diseases of cage and aviary birds. 3rd edition. Baltimore (MD): Williams and Wilkins; 1996. p. 783–94.

[47] Skirnisson K. Mortality associated with renal and intestinal coccidiosis in juvenile eiders in Iceland. Parasitologia 1997;39(4):325–30.

[48] Lowenstein LJ, Petrak ML. Microsporidiosis in two peach-faced lovebirds. In: Midgaki G, Montali RJ, editors. The comparative pathology of zoo animals. Washington (DC): Smithsonian Institution; 1980. p. 365–8.

[49] Poonacha KB, William PD, Stamper RD. Encephalitizoonosis in a parrot. J Am Vet Med Assoc 1985;186(7):700–2.

[50] Randall CJ, Higgins RJ, Harcourt-Brown NH. Microsporidian infection in lovebirds (Agapornis sp.). Avian Pathol 1986;15(2):223–31.

[51] Barton CE, Phalen DN, Snowden KF. Prevalence of microsporidian spores shed by asymptomatic lovebirds: evidence for a potential emerging zoonosis. J Avian Med Surg 2003; 17(4):197–202.

[52] Pulparampil N, Graham D, Phalen D. *Encephalitozoon hellem* in two eclectus parrots (*Eclectus roratus*): identification from archival tissues. J Eukaryot Microbiol 1998;45(6): 651–5.

[53] Degernes LA. Toxicities in waterfowl. Seminars in Avian and Exotic Pet Medicine 1995;4(1):15–22.

[54] Klein PN, Charmatz K, Langenberg J. The effect of flunixin meglumine (Banamine) on the renal function in northern bobwhite quail (*Colinus virginianus*): an avian model. In: Association of Avian Veterinarians Annual Conference Proceedings. Boca Raton (FL): Association of Avian Veterinarians; 1994. p. 128–31.

[55] O'Rourke K. Veterinary drug kills vultures abroad. J Am Vet Med Assoc 2004;224(8):1238, 1240.

[56] Frazier DL, Jones MP, Orosz SE. Pharmacokinetic considerations of the renal system in birds: part II. Review of drugs excreted by renal pathways. J Avian Med Surg 1995;9(2): 104–21.

[57] Flammer K, Clark CH, Drewes LA, et al. Adverse effects of gentamicin in scarlet macaws and galahs. Am J Vet Res 1990;51(3):404–7.

[58] Fernandez-Repollet E, Rowley J, Schwartz A. Renal damage in gentamicin-treated lanner falcons. J Am Vet Med Assoc 1987;181(11):1392–4.

[59] Pollock CG, Carpenter JW, Antinoff N. Birds. In: Carpenter JW, editor. Exotic animal formulary. 3rd edition. St. Louis (MO): Elsevier Saunders; 2005. p. 135–344.

[60] Mollenhauer HH, Corrier DE, Huff WE, et al. Ultrastructure of hepatic and renal lesions in chickens fed aflatoxin. Am J Vet Res 1989;50(5):771–7.

[61] Morgulis MS, Oliveira GH, Dagli ML, et al. Acute 2,4-dichlorophenoxyacetic acid intoxication in broiler chicks. Poult Sci 1998;77(4):509–15.

[62] Kinde H. A fatal case of oak poisoning in a Double-Wattled Cassowary (*Casuarius casuarius*). Avian Dis 1988;32(4):849–51.

[63] Petrak ML. Poisoning and other causalities. In: Petrak ML, editor. Diseases of cage and aviary birds. Philadelphia: Lea & Febiger; 1982. p. 646–52.

[64] Dennis PM, Bennett RA. Ureterotomy for removal of two ureteroliths in a parrot. J Am Vet Med Assoc 2000;217(6):865–8.

[65] Austic RE, Cole RK. Impaired renal clearance of uric acid in chickens having hyperuricemia and articular gout. Am J Physiol 1972;223(3):525–30.

[66] Mallinson ET, Rothenbacher H, Wideman RF, et al. Epizootiology, pathology, and microbiology of an outbreak of urolithiasis in chickens. Avian Dis 1983;28(1):25–43.

[67] Niznik RA, Wideman RF, Cowen BS, et al. Induction of urolithiasis in single comb white Leghorn pullets: effect on glomerular number. Poult Sci 1985;64(8):1430–7.

[68] Wideman RF Jr, Closser JA, Roush WB, et al. Urolithiasis in pullets and laying hens: role of dietary calcium and phosphorus. Poult Sci 1985;64(12):2300–7.

[69] Kamphues J, Otte W, Wolf P. Effects of increasing protein intake on various parameters of nitrogen metabolism in grey parrots (*Psittacus erithacus erithacus*). Abstracts of the First International Symposium on Pet Bird Nutrition. Hannover (Germany): 1997. p. 118.

[70] Pegram RA, Wyatt RD. Avian gout caused by oosporein, a mycotoxin produced by *Chaetomium trilaterale*. Poult Sci 1981;60(11):2429–40.

[71] Siller WG. Avian nephritis and visceral gout. Lab Invest 1959;8:1319–57.

[72] Chandra M, Singh B, Gupta PP, et al. Clinicopathological, hematological, and biochemical studies in some outbreaks of nephritis in poultry. Avian Dis 1985;29(3): 590–600.

[73] Lumeij JT. Plasma urea, creatinine and uric acid concentrations in response to dehydration in racing pigeons. Avian Pathol 1987;16:377–82.

[74] Fudge AM. Avian clinical pathology—hematology and chemistry. In: Altman RB, Clubb SL, Dorrestein GM, et al, editors. Avian medicine and surgery. Philadelphia: WB Saunders; 1997. p. 142–57.

[75] Lumeij JT, Wolfswinkel J. Tissue enzyme profiles of the budgerigar (*Melopsittacus undulates*) [PhD thesis]. In: Lumeij JT, editor. A contribution to clinical investigative methods for birds with special reference to the racing pigeon (*Columbia livia domestica*). Utrecht: University of Utrecht; 1987. p. 71–7.

[76] Kolmstetter CM, Ramsay EC. Effects of feeding on plasma uric acid and urea concentrations in blackfooted penguins (*Spheniscus demersus*). J Avian Med Surg 2000;14(3):177–9.

[77] Lumeij JT, Remple JD, Remple CJ, et al. Plasma chemistry in Peregrine Falcons (*Falco peregrinus*): reference values and physiologic variations of importance for interpretation. Avian Pathol 1998b;27:129–32.

[78] Dorrestein GM. Physiology of the urogenital system. In: Altman RB, Clubb SL, Dorrestein GM, et al, editors. Avian medicine and surgery. Philadelphia: WB Saunders; 1997. p. 622–5.

[79] Goldstein DL, Skadhauge E. Renal and extrarenal regulation of body fluid composition. In: Whittow GC, editor. Sturkie's avian physiology. 5th edition. San Diego (CA): Academic Press; 2000. p. 265–97.

[80] Braun EJ. Integration of renal and gastrointestinal function. J Exp Zool 1999;283(4–5): 495–9.

[81] Lumeij JT, Westerhof I. The use of water deprivation test for the diagnosis of apparent psychogenic polydipsia in a socially deprived African grey parrot (*Psittacus erithacus erithacus*). Avian Pathol 1988;17(4):875–8.

[82] Palmore WP, Fregly MJ, Simpson CE. Catecholamine-induced diuresis in turkeys. Proc Soc Exp Bio Med 1981;167:1–5.

[83] Halsema WB, Alberts H, De Bruijne JJ, et al. Collection and analysis of urine in racing pigeons (*Columba livia domestica*). Avian Pathol 1988;17(1):221–5.

[84] Hochleitner M. Biochemistries: Urinalysis. In: Ritchie BW, Harrison GJ, Harrison LR, editors. Avian medicine: principles and applications. Lake Worth (FL): Wingers Publishing Inc.; 1994. p. 242–4.

[85] Hofbauer H, Krautwald-Junghanns M-E. Transcutaneous ultrasonography of the avian urogenital tract. Vet Radiol Ultrasound 1999;40(1):58–64.

[86] Hildebrandt TH, Pitra C, Göritz F. Transintestinal ultrasonographic sexing. In: European Association of Avian Veterinarians Annual Conference Proceedings. Jerusalem (Israel): 1995. p. 37–41.

[87] Romagnano A, Heard DJ, Johnson RD, et al. Magnetic resonance imaging of the brain and coelomic cavity of the domestic pigeon (Columba livia domestica). Vet Radiol Ultrasound 1996;37(6):431–40.

[88] Speer BL, Harris D, Murray M, et al. Round table discussion: endoscopic renal biopsy. J Avian Med Surg 1997;11(4):273–8.

[89] Marshall KL, Craig LE, Jones MP, et al. Quantitative renal scintigraphy in domestic pigeons (*Columba livia domestica*) exposed to toxic doses of gentamicin. Am J Vet Res 2003;64(4):453–62.

[90] Radin MJ, Hoepf TM, Swayne DE. Use of a single injection solute-clearance method for determination of glomerular filtration rate and effective renal plasma flow in chickens. Lab Anim Sci 1993;43(6):594–6.

[91] Wideman RF, Gregg CM. Model for evaluating avian hemodynamics and glomerular filtration rate autoregulation. Am J Physiol 1988;254(6 Part 2):R925–32.

[92] Brown S, Sandersen SL. Urinary system. In: Kahn CM, Line S, editors. The Merck veterinary manual. Non-infectious diseases of the urinary system in small animals. 9th edition. Summerset: John Wiley & Sons; 2005. p. 1249–88.

[93] Brown SA, Finco DR, Brown CA. Is there a role for dietary polyunsaturated fatty acid supplementation in canine renal disease? J Nutr 1998;128:2765S–7S.

[94] Bauer JE, Markwell PJ, Rawlings JM, et al. Effects of dietary fat and polyunsaturated fatty acids in dogs with naturally developing chronic renal failure. J Am Vet Med Assoc 1999; 215(11):1588–91.

[95] Lumeij JT, Redig PT. Hyperuricemia and visceral gout induced by allopurinol in red-tailed hawks (*Buteo jamaicensis*). In: Proceedings Tagung der Fachgruppe Gefluegelkrankheiten, Giessen, Germany: Deutsche Veterinaermedizinische Gesellschaft; 1992.

[96] Braun EJ. Comparative renal function in reptiles, birds and mammals. Seminars in Avian and Exotic Pet Medicine 1998;7(2):62–71.

[97] Anadón A, Martinez-Larranaga MR, et al. Pharmacokinetics and residues of ciprofloxacin and its metabolites in broiler chickens. Res Vet Sci 2001;71(2):101–9.

[98] Poffers J, Lumeij JT, Redig PT. Investigations into the uricolytic properties of urate oxidase in a granivorous (*Columba livia domestica*) and in a carnivorous (*Buteo jamaicensis*) avian species. Avian Pathol 2002;31(6):573–9.

[99] Bauck L. A clinical approach to neoplastic disease in the pet bird. Seminars in Avian and Exotic Pet Medicine 1994;1(2):65–72.

[100] Macwhirter P, Pyke D, Wayne J. Use of carboplatin in the treatment of renal adenocarcinoma in a budgerigar. Exotic DVM 2002;4(2):11–2.

[101] Machado C, Mihm F, Buckley DN, et al. Disintegration of kidney stones by extracorporeal shockwave lithotripsy in a penguin. In: Proceedings of the First International Conference on Zoological and Avian Medicine. Oahu (Hawaii): 1987. p. 343–9.

**ELSEVIER
SAUNDERS**

**VETERINARY
CLINICS**

Exotic Animal Practice

Vet Clin Exot Anim 9 (2006) 129–159

Renal Pathology in Reptiles

Peernel Zwart, DVM, PhD, DECVP

*Department of Veterinary Pathology, State University,
Yalelaan 1, 358CL Utrecht, The Netherlands*

The class of Reptilia varies widely. It contains:

Squamata (lizards and snakes)
   Sauria: approximately 3000 species
   Serpentes: approximately 2700 species
Chelonia (turtles, tortoises, box turtles): 230 species
Crocodylia (crocodiles, alligators, caimans, gharials): 23 species
Rhynchocephala (tuatara): 1 species

Both the gross morphology and microscopic anatomy of the kidneys are specific for each species. In each species of reptile, the physiology of the renal system has adapted to the specific conditions of life, including, among other factors, the type of food, environmental temperature, and the availability of water. For example, the food may be soft and rich in water (like aquatic plants) or hard and dry (like desert plants).

Reptiles have to adapt to temporary variations in temperature and availability of food. Temperature and behavior are closely connected and are important for normal activity and water homeostasis. The availability of water varies among species. Sea turtles and terrapins (water turtles) live in fairly stable situations. Other reptiles have to cope with wider seasonal variations. Reptiles living in moderate climatic zones are exposed to spring, summer, autumn, and winter periods and must adapt to changes in the availability of food, light, and heat. During cold periods, reptiles may go into hibernation. Some species like the Horsfield's tortoise (*Testudo horsfieldii*) take a "summer rest" during the hottest period of the year. In monsoon-governed climates, the availability of food and water may be quite different. The desert climate is an extreme environment.

The physical features of kidneys, and more especially the glomeruli, reflect the availability of water. This adaptation is especially seen in chelonians. The

E-mail address: bibliozoo.p.zwart@planet.nl

doi:10.1016/j.cvex.2005.10.005
vetexotic.theclinics.com

glomerular tuft is relatively rich in blood capillaries in the Emydae (eg, the red-eared slider, *Trachemys scripta elegans*), which live where water is abundant. In testudines (tortoises) living in a dry environment, the mesangial center is pronounced, and the number of blood capillaries is low.

Reptiles are the first vertebrates to have developed an amnion. The amniotic fluid "replaces" the water in which the embryo develops. Thus, it allows reptilian (and avian) eggs to be laid on land. The period of embryonal development in an egg requires a fundamental adaptation of the metabolism. This adaptation is most obvious in reptiles producing a hard-shelled egg. In these species, the waste products of protein metabolism must be minimally toxic to ensure survival of the embryo. In addition, wastes should be stored as a minimal volume. Uric acid fits these demands. Uric acid is excreted mainly through the proximal segment of the renal tubules as a solid, nontoxic waste, unlike urea found in mammals.

The pathology of the kidneys in reptiles has been poorly studied, but in recent years a number of investigators have specifically studied reptilian renal pathology [1–4].

Necropsy examination of the kidneys

Examination of the kidneys should be based on the normal anatomic situation. Attention is paid to changes in color, inflammatory foci, urate tophi, and urate stasis in collecting ducts. Congenital defects (eg, absence of structures or differences in size and shape between the two kidneys) should be noticed.

In very young animals, the kidneys may be involved in the production of blood cells. In chelonia, the kidneys are rounded to spindle-shaped. In the normal situation, the surfaces are convoluted, much like a folded ribbon. The sharp edges of the ribbon are on the surface of the kidneys. With parenchymal swelling or inflammation, these "edges" bulge. In addition, the nephrogenic zones are situated in these "edges." In subacute or chronic nephritis, the "edges" are even more pronounced. In some chronic cases, the marked proliferation of the nephrogenic zones may give the kidneys a knobby appearance.

In snakes, the right kidney is situated more cranially than the left kidney. The kidneys are elongate and segmented and look somewhat like a sausage cut in slices. The ureter, renal artery, and renal vein run along the visceral surface. In snakes, the sexual segments are situated at the surface of the kidneys. When active, they can be confused with tubules overfilled with urates. Thus a differentiation between active sexual segments, urate stasis, and even gout should be made.

The anatomy can differ in different species of lizard. A misleading situation is seen in chameleons. The sexual segments are localized in clusters, distributed throughout the kidney. In general, these clusters are wedge shaped and can be confused with inflammatory foci.

In lizards (Sauria), the kidneys are situated in the pelvic area [5]. The two kidneys together are triangular in shape. In many species they are fused at the caudal part and may proceed caudally to the cloaca.

Particularly important is the sex of the animal under examination. In male snakes and lizards, the last part of the nephron, before it enters into the collecting duct, is the "sexual segment." This segment proliferates synchronous to the activity of the epididymus. It then enlarges and can be visualized with the naked eye [6]. The enlargement is caused by the whitish secretum accumulating as fine granules in the epithelial cells [7,8].

A urinary bladder is absent in snakes and crocodilians. Chelonids and several lizards (especially iguanids) possess a bladder.

Frequency of renal diseases in reptiles

The frequency of reported renal diseases varies with the technique used to detect it. Based on post mortem examinations and histopathology, the incidence of renal diseases varies between 9.7% (in tortoises) and 11% (in terrapins and turtles) [9,10]. In a general survey concerning routine post mortem material, renal disease was diagnosed in 14% of the reptilian cases [11]. In a specifically directed histopathologic study of 538 kidneys originating from chelonians, snakes, lizards, and a few crocodiles, lesions were observed in 65% of the samples [3]. Routine serologic examination of 1086 European tortoises (Hermann's tortoise [*Testudo hermanni*], spur-thighed tortoise [*T graeca*], marginated tortoise [*T marginata*], and Afghan tortoise [*T horsfieldii*]) delivered as patients to a University of Munich clinic revealed that 26% had nephropathies. Decisive parameters were hyperuricemia (>4 mg/dL) and hypercalcemia in combination with hyperphosphatemia (Ca > 10 mg/dL and P > 5 mg/dL) [12]. Ultrasound examination of 26 tortoises revealed renal disease in 7 animals (27%) [13].

Congenital abnormalities of the kidneys in reptiles

Agenesis/hypoplasia

Agenesis of a kidney has been recorded in a Javan wart snake (*Acrochordus granulatus*) [14] and a western diamondback rattlesnake (*Crotalus atrox*) [2]. In both specimens, the right kidney was absent.

Hypoplasia is noted as very small kidneys. Renal hypoplasia could be recognized only by light microscopy in two Hermann's tortoises. Both had a weak carapace [15].

The author has noted a small extra kidney caudal to the right kidney in an anaconda (*Eunectes murinus*) (Fig. 1) with two otherwise normal kidneys. The third kidney had a normal connection to the ureter and was normal histologically.

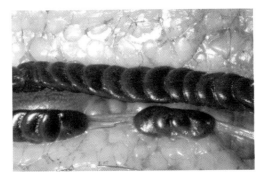

Fig. 1. Anaconda (*Eunectes murinus*) with a small extra kidney situated caudal to the right kidney.

Renal cysts

Renal cysts may occur singly or in a small group or involve the entire kidney (Fig. 2). Especially in the third situation, both kidneys may be affected and show variable degrees of enlargement; clinical consequences can be serious. The author has seen a Yemen chameleon (*Chamaeleo calyptratus*) with pronounced renal cysts that diffusely affected both kidneys. There was a resulting visible distension of the abdomen and compression with cloacal obstruction. Renal and hepatic cysts may be combined, as was found in a giant tegu (*Tupinambis merianae*, previously *T teguixin*) [2]. This latter association has been reported in humans since 1925 [16].

Renal cysts are relatively frequent, especially in European chelonids. They occur sporadically, but in one clutch of 12-month-old Hermann's tortoises two animals had bilateral cystic kidneys [15].

The tubules and eventually the Bowman's spaces are dilated in cystic kidneys. Also, the tubular epithelium becomes flattened. There are occasionally signs of regeneration with focal accumulations of nuclei. The amount of

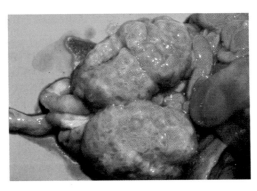

Fig. 2. Black-breasted leaf turtle (*Geoemyda spengleri*) with cystic nephritis.

interstitial tissue is variable but is generally relatively small. There often is no distinct inflammatory infiltration, but secondary gout tophi may develop, which are then surrounded by inflammatory cells.

Renal dysplasia

The author found malformed and underdeveloped glomerulus in a red-eared turtle (Fig. 3) and a Hermann's tortoise. In both cases, only a restricted area of the kidney was altered. Both animals had comparable lesions: enlarged Bowman's spaces that had deformed glomeruli. Although some of the glomeruli were normal, other glomeruli consisted of only a small group of a few capillary loops without recognizable arterioles. The impression was that abnormal glomeruli were still being produced in the connected nephrogenic zone.

Hypervascularity of glomeruli

The author observed a few glomeruli in a Hermann's tortoise with two or even more vasa afferentia (which bring blood to the glomerulus) and vasa efferentia (which take blood away from the glomerulus). Each of the vasa afferentia supplied blood to a deformed tuft of capillaries. Several of these tufts were conglomerated within one Bowman's capsule.

Miscellaneous alterations

The author has noted ciliated epithelial metaplasia in the proximal renal segment in several reptile species. It was distinguished from epithelium in the neck and intermediate segments of the renal tubules, both of which have a smaller diameter and cuboidal epithelial cells with long cilia.

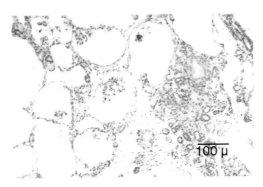

Fig. 3. Red-eared turtle (*Trachemys scripta elegans*) with renal dysplasia (hematoxylin and eosin stain). Bar, 100 μm.

Dilatation of particular tubule segments occurs occasionally without any indication of a cause. The author has seen this dilatation in the renal tubule neck segment of a panther chameleon (*Furcifer pardalis*), the proximal segment of a Hermann's tortoise, and the collecting ducts of a garter snake (*Thamnophis* sp). This type of dilatation differs from congestion of urates in that the remnants of spherules were not present in the noted species.

Arteriolar proliferation was noticed in a Columbian slider (*Trachemys scripta callirostris*). Conglomerates of arterioles were especially present near glomerular vascular poles and the nephrogenic zones. The endothelium of these arterioles had proliferated.

Nephrosis/nephritis

Histopathology of the nephron

Glomeruli

Glomerulonephritis. Although the terms are often used interchangeably, glomerulonephritis specifically implies inflammation of the glomerulus, whereas glomerulopathy is a more general term and indicates any glomerular disease.

According to one survey, acute glomerulonephritis occurred in approximately 27% of the kidneys examined [3]. In these cases, the tuft may completely fill the Bowman's space. A characteristic finding is moderate thickening of the basal glomerular capillary membranes caused by a deposition of a hyaline periodic acid Schiff (PAS)–positive material. In some cases, hyaline material is also located in the mesangium (the center of the glomerulus, which consists of connective tissue mixed with reticulin fibers). The amount of mesangium may increase by mild cellular proliferation. The podocytes may proliferate or swell moderately. In isolated cases, cloudy swelling or accumulations of hyaline droplets may be present in the podocytes. In spite of the low blood pressure and the thickness of the podocytes, a proteinaceous deposit can be present in the Bowman's space.

The outer Bowman's membrane epithelium may swell and proliferate along with hyaline thickening of its basal membrane. The glomerular tuft may adhere to the outer Bowman's capsule. In a number of these cases, the tubules are slightly dilated and may contain hyaline cylinders. The interstitium is incidentally invaded by heterophils.

Acute glomerulonephritis can be divided into a number of subtypes.

Membranous glomerulonephritis occurs with (marked) thickening of the basal capillary membranes (Fig. 4). There are no signs of mesangial cell proliferation, tubule alteration, or invasion of inflammatory cells.

Exudative glomerulonephritis is characterized by the presence of homogenous eosinophilic, Mallory-positive material in the Bowman's spaces and the tubular lumina [4].

Mesangial proliferative glomerulonephritis occurs with proliferation, especially of the cellular elements of the mesangium, although the tuft is not

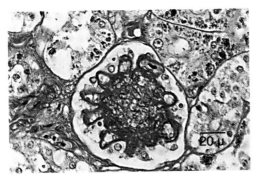

Fig. 4. Boa (*Boa constrictor*) with membranous glomerulonephritis. Notice the position of the nuclei of the podocytes between the capillary loops (periodic acid–Schiff stain). Bar, 20 μm.

distinctly enlarged. There is no deposition of hyaline material or invasion of inflammatory cells [3].

In intracapillary glomerulonephritis, there is a distinct narrowing of the blood capillaries. Intracapillary glomerulonephritis may progress to sclerosis. Accompanying tubular changes are frequent. Gout tophi may develop in the tubules and eventually in the tufts.

Extracapillary glomerulonephritis is characterized by a deformation of glomeruli and an increase in the periglomerular connective tissue. The glomeruli may be surrounded by newly produced connective tissue. These features have also been designated as "basement membrane disease" [17]. In the extracapillary form, there is periglomerular and mesangial fibrosis. The blood capillaries are intact.

Chronic glomerulonephritis is characterized by fibrosis and finally glomerular tuft sclerosis. The blood capillaries are narrow and thickened. Splitting of the basal membranes may occur, and the inner and outer Bowman's capsule may fuse locally.

As occurs in mammals, atrophy of tubules is a rare phenomenon in reptiles, perhaps because the branches of the renal portal system anastomose with the vasa efferentia and surround the tubules. Even with glomerulopathies, the sexual segments may be normally active.

Incidental cases

In *Haemogregarine* sp infection, schizonts may be present in the endothelial cells of glomerular capillaries but cause no disease.

Vitellin, originating from ruptured secondary follicles in the ovary, may be localized in glomerular capillaries and eventually in the Bowman's spaces.

Circulating parasites such as Microfilaria and trophozoites of *Entamoeba invadens* may be found in the capillaries of the tufts. Trophozoites of *Entamoeba invadens* may also enter the Bowman's space. These parasites are discussed more fully in the section on infectious renal diseases: protozoa.

Glomerular lesions, which are related to a more specific pathology, are mentioned under the relevant headings.

Tubular disease

Tubulonephrosis

Tubular nephrosis is defined simply as any degenerative condition of the renal tubules and can be further divided into acute, vacuolating, necrotic, and chronic tubulonephrosis.

Acute tubulonephrosis. In cases of acute tubulonephrosis, the epithelia, especially the proximal segment, are eosinophilic and swollen. Occasionally, mitochondrial swelling can be recognized as central displacement of the nuclei and parallel striping of the cell protoplasm. This "parallel striping" is caused by the swollen mitochondria, which are situated perpendicular to the basement membrane. Some vacuolation may be present. Hyalin droplets may be present in tubular epithelial cells [3].

Such lesions can be found in cases of gentamicin toxicity. The author has also observed these changes in young eastern Hermann's tortoises (*T h boettgeri*) that died spontaneously during hibernation with an acute bacterial glandular gastritis. The author also noted these lesions in a case of acute tubulonephrosis coinciding with bacterial sepsis in a royal python (*Python regius*).

Vacuolating tubulonephrosis. Vacuolation in tubular cells may occur both in the proximal and distal segments of the tubules. It can be combined with some tubule-cell necrosis. Dilatation of the tubular lumina is an accompanying aspect. Some interstitial edema may be present. Vacuolation of renal tubular epithelial cells occasionally coincides with fatty degeneration of the liver. Recognized causative agents are turpentine and insecticides [3]. Metabolic disturbances leading primarily to fatty degeneration of the liver may also be involved.

Necrotic tubulonephrosis. In necrotic tubulonephrosis the majority of the tubular epithelial cells are necrotic. Histologically, the epithelial cells are pale, the protoplasm is mottled, only pyknotic nuclei or fragments of nuclei are visible, and the cell borders are vague. The glomeruli remain intact [3].

Chronic tubulonephrosis. Chronic tubulonephrosis may occur at any age. The author has noted chronic tubulonephrosis in reptiles at hatch and older, making it difficult to place a timeline on the development of this finding. It is especially common in iguanids. In the green (*Iguana iguana*) and black iguana (*Ctenosaura acanthura*), chronic tubulonephrosis occurs mainly in animals 4 to 6 years old. Changes are diffuse, and although the glomeruli are normal, the renal tubules have shortened cells, poorly differentiated epithelium, and a wide lumen (Fig. 5).

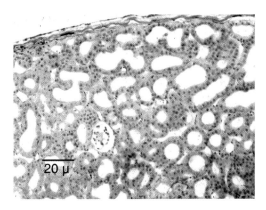

Fig. 5. Green iguana (*Iguana iguana*) with tubulonephrosis. Moderately widened luminal covered with poorly differentiated perihelium (Elastica van Gieson stain). Bar, 20 μm.

Chronic tubulonephrosis leads to a disturbance of the calcium metabolism with metastatic calcium deposition in the large blood vessels and in many organs (liver, lungs, stomach).

Interstitial nephritis

Interstitial nephritis can be divided into acute, subacute, and chronic disease.

In acute interstitial nephritis, there are accumulations of heterophilic granulocytes, lymphocytes, and, rarely, plasma cells. These infiltrations can be monotypic or variable mixtures of the components. Cellular casts may be present in the lumina.

In subacute interstitial nephritis, there is an increase in interstitial connective tissue and marked cellular infiltration. The cellular infiltration may be diffuse or more localized. Some distortion and loss of tubule differentiation may occur.

In chronic interstitial nephritis, there is a marked increase in connective tissue, but the infiltration of inflammatory cells has largely diminished. The distortion of tubuli can be marked. Tubular lumina may range in size from near-normal diameter to excessively dilated. The epithelium, in general, is poorly differentiated. Atrophy of tubules occurs, which may result in the formation of groups of glomeruli. Proteinaceous material may be deposited in the lumina.

Tubulonephrosis may be the initial lesion and is commonly noted with interstitial nephritis. Tubulonephrosis is reflected by irregular distribution and size of epithelial nuclei and variation in the height of the epithelium, with denser groups of nuclei in the higher epithelium.

Subtype: giant cell nephritis

In snakes, the author has seen a few cases of markedly enlarged, pale kidneys (Fig. 6). These kidneys were large enough to be detected by external

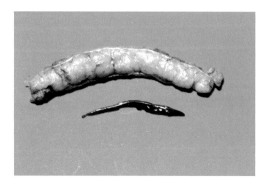

Fig. 6. Corn snake (*Elaphe guttata*) with giant cell nephritis. For comparison, a normal kidney from a healthy corn snake is shown.

inspection as a swelling of the body in the area where the kidneys are situated. This condition is most commonly noted in elaphid snakes. It is characterized by diffuse and significant accumulation of multinucleate giant cells in the interstitium.

The tubules remained intact. Ziehl-Neelsen stain for acid-fast microorganisms has been negative. Transmission electron microscopy has not defined a cause.

Pyelonephritis

Reptiles have no renal pelvis and therefore do not develop pyelonephritis. The collecting ducts run through or over the kidney. In snakes, especially, they are located at the visceral surface of the kidneys. Only occasionally does inflammatory cellular infiltration occur more selectively around the collecting ducts.

Metabolic disturbances

The category of metabolic disturbances is an arbitrary grouping. The various metabolic diseases described are separated from renal pathologies because they are not strictly related to specific kidney lesions.

Pigment deposition

Pigment deposition is a frequent finding (occurring in more than 30% of the kidneys observed by the author). On hematoxylin and eosin staining, the pigment is seen as fine, brownish, rounded or angular granules scattered throughout the cytoplasm. The prolonged Ziehl-Neelsen and iron stains are negative. The pigment has been identified as lipofuscin, resulting from the breakdown and absorption of damaged blood cells [18]. Pigment deposition can occur simultaneously and independently from other tubular changes. In severe cases in various reptile species, the author found a few of these granules in the glomerular mesangium, podocytes, and tubular main and, especially, distal segments. The last observation contrasts with reports by other authors, who observed the granules primarily in main segments [3].

Nephrocalcinosis

Nephrocalcinosis occurs in snakes, lizards, and chelonians with a reported frequency of approximately 16% of renal tissue examined [3]. The author has found minimal calcium deposits in a 2-day-old eastern Hermann's tortoise (*T h boettgeri*) suffering from subacute tubulonephrosis showing loss of tubular epithelial cells. The described tortoise also had severe hepatic fatty degeneration, which may have contributed to 1,25 dihydroxy-cholecalciferol deficiency and altered calcium metabolism, resulting in the observed nephrocalcinosis.

Calcium can be deposited anywhere in the kidney including the glomerular mesangium or, more specifically, in the glomerular basement membranes under the podocytes, in tubular epithelium, and in tubular basement membranes. Casts of calcium may block the renal tubules (Fig. 7) [17]. Furthermore, calcium deposits can be observed in the interstitial connective tissue (Fig. 8) and on elastic membranes in renal arteries.

A peculiar phenomenon is a proliferation reaction of tubular epithelium encapsulating calcium deposits. More details are given in the discussion of proliferation and regeneration.

Nephrocalcinosis usually results from some disturbance in calcium metabolism. Multiple causes are likely. Some authors consider nutritional factors, especially vitamin D deficiency [18]. Others have found no association with osteodystrophy or hypovitaminosis D [9].

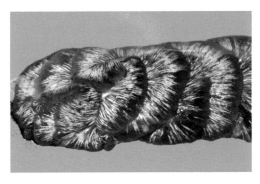

Fig. 7. Boa (*Boa constrictor*) with calcium visibly deposited in renal collecting ducts.

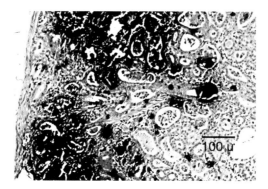

Fig. 8. Red-eared turtle (*Trachemys scripta elegans*) with extensive calcium depositions in the kidney (Kossa stain). Bar, 100 μm.

Renal gout

The frequency of renal gout in a cohort of 538 reptiles subjected to necropsy was found to be around 16% [3].

In reptiles, uric acid is the main end product of both cellular and nuclear proteins in the body. As early as 1850, it was proven that uric acid is quantitatively the most important constituent of urine in the python [19]. Most likely related to the animal's habitat, reptiles excrete various amounts of uric acid, urea, allantoin, and even ammonia through the droppings. It has been demonstrated that in the green turtle (*Chelonia mydas*) ammonia is the most important end phase of protein metabolism, and uric acid is excreted only in small amounts [20]. In snakes and lizards, uric acid is the main component of urine. Uric acid makes up to 83% and 93%, respectively, of totally excreted products in the Hermann's tortoise and emerald lizard (*Lacerta viridis*) [21]. Uric acid is excreted primarily thorough active secretion by the proximal tubules of the kidney. In the green iguana only 6% of uric acid is excreted through the glomerulus, and the remainder is excreted by tubular secretion [22].

Gout occurs in cases of hyperuricemia caused by renal dysfunction. There are always renal lesions preceding the deposition of uric acid in crystalline form in tissues. In early renal gout cases, the remnants of the elongate uric acid crystals deposited in individual proximal segment epithelial cells can be seen histologically in formalinized tissues. Formalin will dissolve uric acid in tissues leaving only a crystal ghost. Gradually, uric acid crystals accumulate around these crystallization centers. Uric acid crystals then may break through the basal membrane of the tubule (seen in PAS-stained slides). At this point, an inflammatory reaction starts, and the characteristic urate tophus is produced. In the typical form, urate tophi consist of radially arranged uric acid crystals surrounded by inflammatory cells (Fig. 9). The inflammation consists of macrophages, some giant cells, variable numbers of heterophilic granulocytes, and some lymphocytes. The numbers of

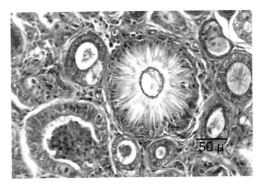

Fig. 9. A characteristic urate tophus in renal tissue (periodic acid–Schiff stain). Bar, 50 µm.

heterophils and lymphocytes vary with the exact nature of the uric acid compound. Under specific circumstances, such as in a cystic kidney, accumulations of uric acid crystals can be found in the tubular lumen, surrounded by proliferated tubular epithelial cells and fixed to the tubular wall with a stem of connective tissue (Fig. 10). In nondilated tubules, several clusters of uric acid may be found close together and may block the lumen.

Tophi may be found distributed throughout the kidney, in the interstitium, or occasionally in the mesangium of glomeruli.

Hypertrophic osteopathy has been suggested to be a serious complication of gout in the green iguana [23].

Other renal deposits

Reptilian renal tissue may accumulate other compounds.

Deposition of amyloid has rarely been mentioned. In a Central American boa (*Boa constrictor imperator*) and a rainbow water snake (*Enhydris*

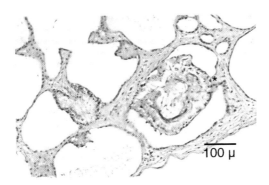

Fig. 10. Yemen chameleon (*Chamaeleo calyptratus*). Gout tophus produced on a small area of some damaged epithelial cells. A "stem" (*) connects the tophus to the interstitial tissue. A second tophus extends in two adjoining tubules. Proliferated epithelial cells cover the tophi (hematoxylin and eosin stain). Bar, 100 µm.

enhydris), deposition of material, the tinctorial qualities of which were comparable to mammalian amyloid, was reported [17]. An amyloid-like deposition has been described in the renal interstitium and mesangium of glomeruli in four Komodo dragons (*Varanus komodoensis*). This material stained amphophilic with Congo red but was not birefringent; it did not stain with crystal violet, PAS, or Von Kossa stains [24]. In a specifically directed study of hyaline glomerular changes in reptiles that included the aid of electron microscopy, amyloid was not detected [25].

Proteins in the form of *Leishmania agamae* promastigote antigens were detected in renal epithelial cells by the use of an immunoperoxidase technique [26]. Heavy metals can accumulate in the kidneys. Substantial amounts of cadmium were found in the kidneys of red-eared turtles following intraperitoneal injection with 10 mg cadmium/d for 6 days [27]. Brown house snakes (*Lamprophis fuliginosus*) were exposed to 10 and 20 μg selenium/g body weight by injecting seleno-D,L-methionine into their prey. Significant concentrations were accumulated in the kidneys (and other organs) when exposed to these high doses [28]. Mercury can also be accumulated in the kidneys as reported in American alligators (*Alligator mississippiensis*) [29].

Infectious renal diseases

Helminths

Nematoda

Nematode infections of the kidneys in reptiles are rare. One case of severe parasitic nephritis and ureteritis in a Burmese python (*Python molurus bivittatus*) has been described. The strongyloides species involved resembled *Strongyloides gulae*, a parasite of snakes, which normally lives in the esophagus [30].

Filaria (microfilaria)

Microfilaria can be found in the circulating blood in all renal blood vessels, including arteries, veins, and capillaries of the glomerular tufts. Pathologic changes related to microfilaria have not been observed.

Trematoda

Trematodes infecting exclusively the kidneys are known especially in boas and pythons. In the boa constrictor, the flukes *Styphlodora horrida* [31,32], *S condita*, and a larger number of small trematodes can be found in the kidney [33]. In pythons, *S renalis* exclusively inhabits the ureter [34]. *S horrida* lives in both the ureter and the larger collecting ducts. Collecting ducts containing parasites are enlarged and filled with urates, eggs, debris of the parasites, and some calcium deposits in boa constrictors. The renal epithelial lining was locally damaged, multinucleate giant cell reaction was present, and there was an increase in connective tissue around the affected areas. The interstitial reaction led to glomerular and tubular atrophy.

The trematodes do not completely block the ureter. Desquamation of epithelial cells and acute cellular infiltration may be noted where the ventral suckers of the flukes attach to the epithelium. Mushroom-shaped protrusions of proliferated epithelium may also be found. The surrounding interstitial connective tissue may proliferate at sites of more extensive epithelial damage and may lead to a thickening of the ureteral wall [35]. With unilateral infection, the affected kidney may atrophy, while the contralateral kidney hypertrophies. In a python seen by the author, the weights of the ipsilateral and contralateral kidney were 17 g and 93 g, respectively (Fig. 11).

The small spirorchiid trematodes mentioned previously may be found diffusely in the renal tubules. They may cause a local dilatation of the tubule and flattening of the epithelium [33].

In freshwater terrapins (*T s elegans, Chrysemys picta* [36], *Emys orbicularis*, and others) and saltwater turtles, eggs of spirorchiid trematodes may be found in renal tissue. The author has seen trematode eggs spread throughout the body in numerous oceanic turtle species. Eggs may be found in connection with granulomatous reactions in renal tissue in green turtles [37]. Granulomatous lesions in the kidneys and elsewhere were noted in black turtles (*Chelonia mydas agassizii*) infected with the trematode *Learedius learedi* [38].

Protozoa

Spironucleus (synonym: Hexamita)

Hexamita parva (Alexieff 1912) is primarily an intestinal parasite, but it has been recognized as a diplomonad flagellate invading the kidneys, especially of terrapins (water turtles) and less commonly of chelonians

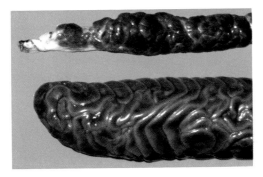

Fig. 11. Python (unknown species). Unilateral trematodes infection in a kidney. The larger kidney weighed 93 g (normal); the atrophied kidney weighed 17 g.

(tortoises). In water turtles, the disease tends to be subacute. In chelonians, spironucleus infection can persist over many years. The author has noted such a chronic case (at least 8 years' duration) in a yellow-footed tortoise (*Geochelone denticulata*).

At post mortem examination, bands on the surface of affected kidneys may be slightly enlarged and show a distinct swelling in water turtles. Metastatic calcification may result from a secondary disturbance of calcium metabolism in chronically infected tortoises. The most pronounced lesions are seen in the superficial portion of the kidneys and in and around the collecting ducts. Sometimes there is epithelial destruction. In affected dilated tubules, hyaline casts or invasion of mostly heterophilic inflammatory cells may occur. Glomerular lesions are frequent. Proliferation of the visceral layer of the Bowman's capsule is sometimes noted. Other lesions include thickening of the glomerular tuft capillary basement membranes.

A more generalized chronic interstitial nephritis may occur with chronicity. Distension and distortion of tubules and deposition of calcium in tubular epithelium and interstitium may be noted.

Spironuclei flagellates can be found in the tubules (Fig. 12), again near the renal surface. The parasites are seen as small, oval-shaped forms with anterior-situated nuclei. Normally the two nuclei cannot be seen apart. The flagellae can be recognized in well-stained slides. The parasites stain particularly well with Heidenhain's iron alum hematoxylin stain [40].

Entamoeba

The protozoa are now usually regarded as a separate kingdom divided into seven phyla, three of which occur in the kidneys of reptiles.

Entamoeba invadens

Entamoeba invadens is a well-known reptile pathogen primarily affecting the intestinal tract. This amoeba is able to infect snakes, lizards, and

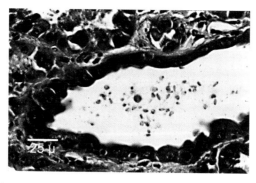

Fig. 12. Red-eared turtle (*Trachemys scripta elegans*) with *Hexamita parva* in a renal tubule (Heidenhain's iron alum hematoxylin stain). Bar, 25 μm.

chelonians. The optimal temperature for multiplication and pathogenic activity is 73.4° to 82.4°F (23°–28°C). An exceptional case of generalized amoebiasis has been reported in a tuatara (*Sphenodon punctatus*), which lives at temperatures as low as 55.4°F (13°C) [41]. Amoebiasis has also been described in captive sea turtles [42].

With generalized infections, extensive areas of renal necrosis may occur. The amoebae are found specifically in the outer necrobiotic zone around the lesion in the kidney. Depending on the type and number of bacteria coming from the intestinal tract (secondary infection) and present in the renal lesions, inflammatory reactions are variable. In some cases, amoeba may be found in the Bowman's spaces or in tubules with no lesions (Fig. 13) [39].

Apicomplexa (coccidia)

Intranuclear stages of coccidia have been found in two juvenile radiated tortoises (*Geochelone radiata*). Animals were anorectic, lethargic, and variably anemic. There was multifocal degeneration of tubular epithelium seen as a granular, pale, eosinophilic cytoplasm. Occasionally, tubules contained amorphous eosinophilic material. There was a marked karyomegaly and intranuclear structures, which resembled inclusion bodies. These intranuclear structures were round to elliptical, eosinophilic to amphophilic forms, often up to 8 μm in diameter. Infected nuclei could be up to two times the normal size with marginated chromatin. With transmission electron microscopy, stages of developing coccidia were distinct. Minimal to moderate interstitial infiltrate consisting of lymphocytes and a few plasma cells was seen [18].

Klossiella boae *(coccidia)*

Klossiella boae has been described in the boa [2,43]. The parasite identified as *Tyzzeria boae* may be the same parasite as *Klossiella boae* [44]. Both parasitize the collecting ducts and eventually the ureter. The various

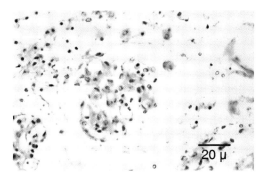

Fig. 13. Garter snake (*Thamnophis sirtalis*) with *Entamoeba invadens* in Bowman's space of the kidney (hematoxylin and eosin stain). Bar, 20 μm.

stages of trophozoites, macro- and microgametocytes, schizonts, and the small coccidia can be found in the renal epithelial cells. Coccidia oocysts may also appear in the renal tubular lumens. This parasite causes little damage. Epithelial cells bearing parasitic stages are swollen and bulge.

Goussia *spp (coccidia)*

Although it is somewhat speculative; it is likely that sporulated oocysts of the coccidium *Goussia* spp were found in the kidneys and several other organs of Nile Crocodiles (*Crocodylus niloticus*) [45].

Myxosporidia

Myxosporidia are protozoa belonging to the class Myxosporea, phylum Myxozoa. One of the key characteristics of Myxosporidia is that all stages, except during sexual reproduction, are multinucleated forms that have enveloping (primary) cells containing enveloped (secondary) cells. Of the Myxosporidia occurring in lower vertebrates, only representatives of the genus *Myxidium* have been reported in the urinary system of chelonians [46,47]. Little is known about their pathogenicity [48,49].

In turtles, *Myxidium mackiei* (Bosanquet 1910) has been described in the kidneys of the Indo-Gangetic soft-shelled turtle (*Trionyx gangeticus*) [48] and Anderson's flap-shelled turtle (*Lissemys punctata andersonii*) [47]. *Myxidium danilewskyi* (Laveran, 1889) has been found in the kidneys of an aged European pond turtle (*Emys orbicularis*) (Mutschmann, personal communication, 2005). An unidentified *Myxidium* species (most probably *M danilewskyi*) has been found in the kidneys of another European pond turtle (author's unpublished data) and in 90% of 60 juvenile male and female Tracaja turtles (*Podocnemis unifilis*) [47].

Macroscopically, affected kidneys may appear pale and swollen. The parasites generally lead to degeneration or necrosis of the renal tubular epithelia and ectasia of the lumina. Throphozoites and spores adhere to the epithelium. Spores may be found free in the urinary bladder.

The author observed throphozoites and pansporoblasts in the parietal (Fig. 14) and visceral epithelium of about 50% of the Bowman's capsules in European pond turtles. About 40% of the renal tubular lumina also contained plasmodium stages with numerous nuclei. Myxosporidian parasites were occasionally present in disrupted epithelial cells, whereas spores were commonly found in collecting ducts. Electron microscopy examination revealed decreased, compressed, or effaced renal tubular microvilli in the turtles infected with *M mackiei* [47]. The interstitial inflammatory reaction may vary from minimal interstitial lymphocytic inflammation (*E orbicularis*), to a chronic interstitial nephritis (*P unifilis*).

Microsporidia

Microsporidia have been observed in renal epithelial cells of the inland bearded dragon (*Pogona vitticeps*). In hematoxylin and eosin–stained

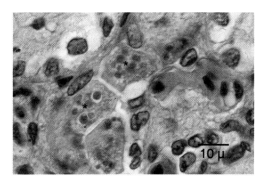

Fig. 14. European pond turtle (*Emys orbicularis*) with trophozoites of Myxidium (*) in the parietal layer of the Bowman's capsule (hematoxylin and eosin stain). Bar, 10 μm.

sections, clusters of lightly basophilic intracytoplasmacytic microorganisms were observed in distended cytoplasmic vacuoles. The microorganism was gram positive and acid-fast positive and had a small polar granule that stained positive with PAS stain. Transmission electron microscopy demonstrated merogonic and sporogonic stages of a protozoan, compatible with members of the phylum Microspora, within cytoplasmic vacuoles in distended renal epithelial cells [50].

Viral infections

Reptilian kidneys are affected by some viruses. With the retroviral inclusion body disease, intracytoplasmic, eosinophilic inclusion bodies can be found in epithelial cells of the proximal and distal renal tubules. The glomerular epithelial cells may contain small numbers of inclusion bodies [51]. In experimentally infected boas, one animal developed glomerulonephritis [52]. Herpesvirus-infected map turtles (*Graptemys pseudogeographica* and *G barbouri*) were noted to have intranuclear inclusions within renal tubule epithelial cells [53].

Bacterial infections

The bacteria reported in reptilian renal infections are predominantly gram negative and are primarily *Pseudomonas* or *Aeromonas* spp [54]. *Vibrio alginolyticus*, *Aeromonas hydrophyla*, and *Flavobacterium* spp were isolated from farmed marine turtles (*C mydas* and *Eretmochelys imbricata*) that had septicemia. Toxic changes were noted in the kidneys [55].

With acute septicemia, the renal blood vessels may be completely blocked by accumulated bacteria (Fig. 15). Also, bacteria may be found in proteinaceous material in the renal tubules [39]. Renal tubular cell degeneration, *Pasteurella piscida*, and *A hydrophyla* septicemia were found during a die off in approximately 4500 farm-raised soft-shelled turtles (*Malaclemys*

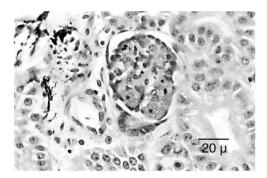

Fig. 15. Mediterranean spur-thighed tortoise (*Testudo graeca ibera*) with glomerular capillaries (*) filled with bacteria (hematoxylin and eosin stain). Bar, 20 μm.

terrapin centrata) [56]. Bacteria may also cause more diffuse heterophilic inflammation. Renal abscesses may also result from bacterial infections.

Spirochetes in the glomeruli were associated with multiple adhesions of the Bowman's membranes in a septicemic Asian box turtle (*Cistoclemmys flavomarginata*, previously *Cuora flavomarginata*) [57]. Experimental infections in snakes and turtles with *Leptospira pomona* induced interstitial nephritis [58].

Streptococcus *species*

Infections with specific alpha-hemolytic, encapsulated gram-positive Streptococci have been found in lizards such as the green anole (*Anolis carolinensis*), girdle-tailed lizard (*Cordylus cordylus*), emerald lizard, wall lizard (*Podarcis muralis*), and house gecko (*Gekko monarchus*) [59,60]. The bacteremia seemed to persist over long periods. Numerous streptococci were found between the erythrocytes in all renal blood vessels. Bacteria were especially distinct with PAS staining. Pathologic lesions were seen as tubular separations, which were incarcerated by masses of bacteria [60].

Mycobacteria

Basic research, using experimental infections, has shown that mycobacterial infections in reptiles share characteristics with those in mammals and birds.

In spontaneous mycobacterial renal infectious, renal granulomas are defined by central necrosis, generally containing large numbers of acid-fast rods, surrounded by multinucleate giant cells (Langerhans' type) and macrophages with a fibrotic capsule. In experimentally infected emerald lizards, mycobacteriosis runs an acute course with a progressive character leading to the production of epithelioid cells [61]. Lizards, crocodiles, snakes [2], and chelonians are all considered susceptible to mycobacteria.

Mycobacterium chelonae has been identified in a Kemp's Ridley sea turtle (*Lepidochelys kempii*) with multifocal arthritis [62]. *Mycobacterium avium* serotype 8 has been isolated from nodules in the kidneys and other organs of a green sea turtle [63].

Fungal infections

Renal fungal infections are generally related to systemic mycoses, and the pathologic changes are variable. *Penicillium griseofulvum* caused whitish nodules consisting of multifocal granulomas with branching hyphae that, in some cases, extended into adjacent parenchyma in Seychelles giant tortoise (*Megalochelys gigantea*) [64].

Ubiquitous fungi such as *Geotrichum candidum* can be part of the resident microflora or act as a pathogen. Fungal elements were seen in areas of cellular necrosis with mild associated inflammation in a giant tortoise (*Geochelone nigra*, previously *Geochelone elephantopus*) [65].

Plant pathogens may incidentally infect turtles and invade the kidneys. A Kemp's Ridley sea turtle developed systemic infection (including the kidneys) with *Colletotrichum acutatum* [66].

Proliferation and regeneration

Neogenic areas or nephrogenic zones are remarkable structures in the reptilian kidney that may undergo proliferation and regeneration.

Groups of small tubules embedded in renal connective tissue were noted as an aspect of the normal microscopic anatomy in the sand lizard (*Lacerta agilis*). These regions were considered to be meta-nephrogenic tissue located at the tips of dichotomously branching intralobular arteries. Pseudoglomeruli were also isolated from the tissue [67]. Comparable structures were found in tortoises [68]. Complete new nephrons were noted in the slow worm (*Anguis fragilis*) [69]. Although originally described in lizards, they are easily recognized during routine histopathology in chelonians and are seen only rarely in lizards.

In cases of subacute and chronic nephritis, the nephrogenic zones can proliferate and produce new nephrons at increased speed. The new nephrons are characteristically embryonic with numerous small cells, basophilic protoplasm, and a relatively large nucleus. Both new glomeruli and tubules can be seen (Fig. 16). In chronic cases, the renal surface can become knobby because of marked proliferation of the nephrogenic zones. It may be noted during histology, especially of chelonians, that the original renal tissue is largely destroyed, and relatively well-organized new renal tissue is present at the periphery (Fig. 17).

Renal tubular epithelia have a remarkable ability to react to foreign substances. This phenomenon is recognized around calcium deposits (Fig. 18) and especially gout tophi present in the renal lobules. In several cases observed by the author, renal epithelial cells were seen encapsulating foreign material by growing around or over it.

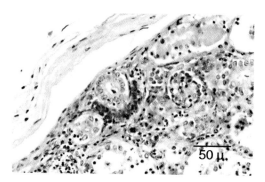

Fig. 16. Hermann's tortoise (*Testudo hermanni*) with an active nephrogenic zone (hematoxylin and eosin stain). Bar, 50 μm.

A more irregular proliferation with metaplasia, indicated by loss of secretory function, may occur when uric acid is precipitated in quantity in the tubules. Vigorous regeneration may block tubular drainage [17].

In an experimental study using wall lizards (*Podarcis siculus* (formerly, *Lacerta sicula*) and sand lizards, the renal tubules were experimentally damaged using mercury bichloride orally at a dose of 20 mg/kg body weight. This dose, which kills mice within 18 hours, provoked a pronounced tubulonephrosis when the wall lizards were kept at 36°C (96.8°F) [2].

The experiments were performed at 36°C (96.8°F) and 26°C (78.8°F). At 36°C, an acute tubulonephrosis, mainly in the proximal segments, developed within 24 hours. The renal epithelial cell brush borders were swollen or even absent. Isolated cells were more severely degenerated (pyknotic nuclei, karyorhexis) or even necrotic during the first week of the experiment. At 26°C, all changes took longer to develop and were less pronounced. Signs of epithelial regeneration, in the form of mitoses and basophilic-staining homogeneous protoplasm, were present at 36°C beginning at 48 hours after

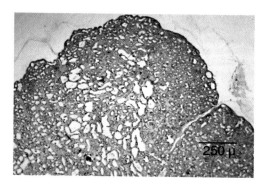

Fig. 17. Leopard tortoise (*Geochelone pardalis*) with a dense outer zone of the kidney in a case of tubulonephrosis. New renal tissue has been produced by the nephrogenic zones (hematoxylin and eosin stain). Bar, 250 μm.

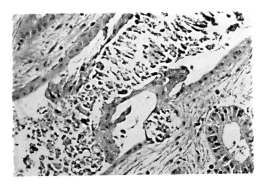

Fig. 18. Boa (*Boa constrictor*) with epithelial proliferation related to deposition of calcium in a renal collecting duct (hematoxylin and eosin stain). Bar, 50 μm.

injection and persisting over the following 8 weeks. In summary, both the degenerative and regenerative processes were more intense at 36°C than at 26°C. The tubular epithelia of animals kept at 36°C had healed after 32 weeks; at 26°C, healing was complete after 64 weeks [2].

Trauma

Renal trauma is rarely noted in reptiles. Obviously, wild animals may suffer from predatory attacks and road traffic injuries. In captivity, such traumas are less common. Severe renal damage caused by an unsecured branch that fell and crushed the pelvis of a captive adult green iguana has been described [5]. Trauma from grass mowers may occasionally involve the kidneys of chelonians.

Tumors

Primary renal tumors are rare in reptiles. Metastatic neoplasia are more likely to be noted in the kidney. Electron microscopy can help identify the type of malignant cells. Electron microscopy was used to identify metastatic squamous cell carcinoma cells as epithelial keratinocytes in the kidneys of two loggerhead turtles (*C caretta*) [70].

Viruses may play a role in the occurrence of renal tumors in reptiles. Leucosis in a boa in the presence of unidentified virus particles has been reported [71]. Type A–like retroviral particles were identified in an emerald tree boa (*Corallus caninus*) suffering from metastatic intestinal adenocarcinoma. Metastases were found in the kidney and other organs. The authors noted that the role of the virions in the origin of the intestinal adenocarcinoma remained uncertain (Table 1) [72].

Vitamin A deficiency

Vitamin A deficiency is known to lead to squamous metaplasia of multiple epithelial structures. Captive terrapins are especially at risk [82].

Table 1
Examples of tumors in reptilian kidneys

Tumor	Animal species
Gastric carcinoma (met) [17]	East african side-neck turtle (*Pelusios subniger*)
Adenocarcinoma [73,74]	Eastern box turtle (*Terrapene carolina*)
Lymphoblastic lymphosarcoma [73]	Hermann's tortoise (*T hermanni*)
Adenocarcinoma [74]	
Lymphoreticular neoplasia [75]	Florida soft shell turtle (*Apalone ferox*)
	(formerly: *Trionyx ferox*)
Myelotic leucosis [76]	African helmeted turtle (*Pelomedusa subrufa*)
Lymphoma [77]	Asian brown tortoise (*Manouria emys*)
	(formerly: *Testudo emys*)
Myxofibroma [78]	Green turtle (*Chelonia mydas*)
Lymphoblastic lymphoma [79]	Loggerhead sea turtle (*Caretta caretta*)
Squamous cell carcinoma (met) [70]	2 Loggerhead sea turtles (*C caretta*)
Leucosis (syst) [71]	Boa (*B constrictor*)
Gastric adenocarcinoma (met) [80]	Eastern indigo snake (*Drymarchon couperi*)
	(formerly: *Drymarchon corais couperi*)
Renal cell carcinoma [81]	Corn snake (*Elaphe guttata*)

Abbreviations: met, metastasis; syst, systemic.

Renal collecting ducts may reveal squamous metaplasia in advanced cases [83].

An exceptional case of vitamin A deficiency occurred in a gharial (*Gavialis gangeticus*) [84]. In this animal, tubular squamous metaplasia progressed to the Bowman's capsules. Locally, hyperkeratosis occurred, which led to the production of epithelial pearls. These changes were combined with deposits of calcium and urates in the tubuli. The interstitial connective tissue had markedly increased.

The author observed a case in a red-eared turtle, in which desquamated cornified cells had accumulated in the renal collecting ducts and led to the formation of large cystic spaces.

Intoxication

Intoxication with the insecticide azinphos-methyl killed snakes and a South African monitor (*Varanus exanthematicus*). Among other findings, parenchymatous degeneration of the renal tubular epithelium was noted [85].

Ureter

The author observed ureteritis in a green tree python (*Morelia viridis*). (Fig. 19) The ureter revealed an irregular proliferation of the epithelium and submucosal lymphocytic and heterophilic inflammation. Many urate tophi were embedded in the perihilar region and were surrounded by proliferated epithelium. In addition, there were numerous urate tophi in the severely altered kidney.

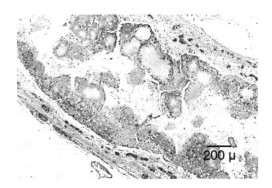

Fig. 19. Green tree python (*Morelia viridis*) with urethritis in a case of gout (hematoxylin and eosin stain). Bar, 200 μm.

Monocercomonas

Monocercomonas sp is a flagellated parasite of the intestinal tract [86]. The author observed ureteritis with dilatation and infiltration of inflammatory cells and large numbers of *Monocercomonas* sp in an unidentified species of snake.

Trematodes

The ureters are the specific location for trematodes (*Styphlodora renalis* and *S horrida*) in the boa and python. The ureter is often dilated and yellowish in color and is filled with parasites, urates, mucus, small amounts of calcium, and cellular debris [87]. There is often chronic inflammation with some cellular infiltration and an increase in connective tissue. Spirorchiid trematodes have also been found in the ureters of a red-eared turtle, which also had ureteroliths [88].

Ureteroliths

Ureteroliths are rare. One case describes bilateral calcium phosphate ureteroliths in a red-eared slider turtle [88].

Urinary bladder

Bladder stones

Urinary bladder stones composed of uric acid are reported especially in lizards such as the green iguana [89,90]. Stones also occur in tortoises [91,92]. Stones in the urinary bladder are not necessarily connected with renal lesions and gout, but the combination has been reported [93].

Eggs

Complete, shelled eggs may enter into the urinary bladder through the cloaca and the short connection between cloaca and bladder in female tortoises and occasionally in iguanas. The specific cause is not known.

Spironucleus

Spironucleus (*H parva*) may invade the urinary bladder from the intestines or cloaca leading to a moderate infiltration of lymphocytes in the wall of the bladder. The urine may become mucinous and turbid with chronic infections. Numerous mucus-producing cells were present in the epithelial lining in some cases observed by the author.

Myxidium

Spores of *Myxidium* spp may be found free in the urine [46,47]. There is no known disease associated with finding these organisms in the urine and kidney tissues.

Trematodes

Monogenetic trematodes such as *Polystomoidella* spp, *Polystomoides* spp, and *Neopolystoma* spp can be found in the urinary bladder of freshwater chelonians [87]. Pathologic changes caused by *Neopolystoma orbiculare* were caused by the presence of eggs in the wall of the urinary bladder of freshwater chelonians. The urinary bladder wall often reveals a diffuse infiltration of eosinophils and lymphocytes. Clusters of eggs were surrounded by granulomas with inflammatory infiltrates consisting of macrophages, lymphocytes, and occasional multinucleate giant cells. In freshwater chelonians, the granulomas formed polyps that projected into the bladder lumen [94].

Eggs of spirorchiid trematodes can be present in the urine, but their significance is unknown [34].

References

[1] Braun LJ. Comparative renal function in reptiles, birds and mammals. Seminars in Avian and Exotic Pet Medicine 1998;7(2):62–71.
[2] Zwart P. Studies on renal pathology of reptiles [doctoral thesis]. Utrecht, The Netherlands: State University; 1963.
[3] Seybold J. Ein Beitrag zur Nierenpathologie bei Reptilien [A contribution to the renal pathology in reptiles] [doctoral thesis]. Munich, Germany: Ludwig-Maximillian University; 1993.
[4] Keunecke S. Vergleich klinischer und pathomorphologischer Befunde bei Nephropathien der Schildkröten [Comparison of clinical and pathomorphologic findings in nephropathies of chelonians] [doctoral thesis]. Hannover, Germany: Veterinary University; 1999.
[5] Hernandez-Divers SJ. Renal disease in the green iguana (*Iguana iguana*): pathogenesis, diagnosis and management [RCVS diploma thesis]. London: Royal College of Veterinary Science; 2000.

[6] Goldberg SR. Reproduction in the coffee snake, *Ninia maculata* (Serpentes: Colubridae), from Costa Rica. Texas J Sci 2004;56(1):81–4.

[7] Regaud C, Policard A. Sur l'existence de diverticules du tube urinipare sans relations avec les corpuscules de Malpighi chez les serpents et sur l'independence relative des fonctions glomérulaire et glandulaire du rein en general [On the existence of diverticles of the renal tubules, with no relation to the Malpighian corpuscles in snakes and on the relative independence of the glomerular and glandular functions of the kidney in general]. CR Hebd Soc Biol 1903;55:1028.

[8] Bishop JE. A histological and histochemical study of the kidney tubule of the common garter snake, *Thamnophis sirtalis*, with special reference to the sexual segment in the male. J Morphol 1959;104:307.

[9] Keymer I. Diseases of chelonians: (1) necropsy survey of tortoises. Vet Rec 1978;103(25): 548–52.

[10] Keymer I. Diseases of chelonians: (2) necropsy survey of terrapins and turtles. Vet Rec 1978; 103(26):577–82.

[11] Bosch H, Frank W. Häufige Erkrankungen bei in Terrarium gehaltenen Amphibien und Reptilien [The most frequent diseases of amphibia and reptiles kept in terraria]. Salamandra (Frankf) 1983;19:29–54.

[12] Kölle P, Hoffmann R. Incidence of renal diseases in tortoise patients. Kleintierpraxis 2002; 47(6):347–55.

[13] Gumpenberger M. Untersuchungen am Harntrakt und weiblichen Genitaltrakt von Schildkröten mit Hilfe bildgebender Technik [Research on the urinary tract and the female genital tract of chelonians, using pictorial techniques] [doctoral thesis]. Vienna, Austria: Veterinary University; 1996.

[14] Bergman RAM. The anatomy of Acrochordinae. Proceedings of the Dutch Academy of Science Series C Biologic and Medical Science 1958;61:145–62.

[15] Haefeli W, Zwart P. Panzerweiche bei jungen Landschildkröten und deren möglichen Ursachen [Weakening of the carapace in young tortoises and the possible causes]. Prakt Tierarzt 2000;81(2):129–32.

[16] Gruber GB. Entwicklungsstörungen der Nieren und Harnleiter [Congenital disorders of kidneys and ureter]. In: Henke F, Lubarsch O, editors. Handbuch der speziellen pathologischen Anatomie und Histologie [Handbook of special pathological anatomy and histology], vol . 6 part 1. Berlin: Springer; 1925. p. 1.

[17] Cowan FD. Diseases of captive reptiles. J Am Vet Med Assoc 1968;153:848–59.

[18] Jacobson E-R, Schumacher J, Telford SR, et al. Intranuclear coccidiosis in radiated tortoises (*Geochelone radiata*). J Zoo Wildl Med 1994;25(1):95–102.

[19] Boussignault M. Recherches sur la quantité d'ammoniaque contenue dans l'urine [Research on the quantity of ammonia in urine]. Annales de Chimie et de Physique 1850;29:472.

[20] Kahlil F. Excretion in reptiles. Non protein nitrogen constituents of the urine of the sea turtle *Chelone mydas*. J Biol Chem 1974;171:611.

[21] Perschmann C. Ueber die Bedeutung der Nierenpfortader insbesondere fuer die Ausscheidung von Harnstoff und Harnsaeure bei *Testudo hermanni* Gml und *Lacerta viridis* Laur. sowie ueber die Funktion der Harnblase bei Lacerta viridis Laur. [Concerning the importance of the renal portal vein, especially in regard of excretion of urea and uric acid in *Testudo hermanni* Gml. and *Lacerta viridis* Laur., as well as the function of the urinary bladder in *Lacerta viridis* Laur.]. Zool Beitr 1956;2:447.

[22] Marshall EK. Kidney secretion in reptiles. Proc Soc Exp Biol Med 1931;29b:971.

[23] Ball RL, Dumonceaux G, MacDonald C. Hypertrophic osteopathy associated with renal gout in a green iguana, *Iguana iguana*. In: Proceedings of the Sixth Annual Conference of the Association of Reptile and Amphibian Veterinarians. Columbus (OH): Association of Reptile and Amphibian Veterinarians; 1999. p. 49–50.

[24] Garner M, Gyimesi ZS, Rasmussen JM, et al. An amyloid-like deposition disorder in Komodo Dragons. In: Proceedings of the Tenth Annual Conference of the Association of

Reptile and Amphibian Veterinarians. Minneapolis (MN): Association of Reptile and Amphibian Veterinarians; 2003. p. 50–1.

[25] Jakob W, Wesemeier H-H. Hyaline renal glomerular changes in reptiles: is there any evidence for amyloidosis? In: Proceedings of the Fifth International Symposium on the Pathology of Reptiles and Amphibians. Alphen aan den Rijn, The Netherlands; 1995. p. 169–72.

[26] Ingram G, Molyneux D. Responses of European green lizards *Lacerta viridis* following administration of *Leishmanis agamae* promastigotes. Vet Parasitol 1984;17(1):1–15.

[27] Thomas P, Baer K, White RB. Isolation and partial characterization of metallothionein in the liver of the red-eared turtle *(Trachemys scripta)* following intraperitoneal administration of cadmium. Comp Biochem Physiol C Pharmacol Toxicol Endocrinol 1994;107(2):221–6.

[28] Hopkins W, Staub AB, Baionno JA, et al. Trophic and maternal transfer of selenium in brown house snakes (*Lamprophis fuliginosus*). Ecotoxicol Environ Saf 2004;58(3):285–93.

[29] Heatonjones TG, Homer BL, Heatonjones DL, et al. Mercury distribution in American alligators *(Alligator mississippiensis)* in Florida. J Zoo Wildl Med 1997;28(1):62–70.

[30] Veazey R, Stewart T, Snider TG. Ureteritis and nephritis in a Burmese python (*Python molurus bivitattus*) due to Strongyloides sp. infection. J Zoo Wildl Med 1994;25(1):119–22.

[31] Kazacos KR, Fisher LF. Renal styphlodoriasis in a boa constrictor. J Am Vet Med Assoc 1977;1(9):876–8.

[32] Chiodini R, Sundberg JP. *Styphlodora horrida* in the kidneys and ureters of a boa constrictor (*Boa constrictor*). Vet Med Small Anim Clin 1980;75:877–8.

[33] Frank W. Infektionen mit Parasiten [Infections with parasites]. In: Isenbügel E, Frank W, editors. Heimtierkrankheiten [Diseases of pet animals]. Basel, Switzerland: Ulmer Verlag; 1985. p. 226–320.

[34] Doton N, Divina B. Helminth parasites of *Python reticulatus* (Schneider). Philippine J Vet Med 1993;30(2):67–70.

[35] Tury E, Kobuley T. Pathological changes caused by trematodes in the urinary system of a boa constrictor. Verh Ber Erkrg Zootiere 1973;15:343–6.

[36] Johnson CA, Griffith JW, Tenorio P, et al. Fatal trematodiasis in research turtles. Cordova (TN): American Association for Laboratory Animal Science; 1998. p. 340–3.

[37] Greiner E, Forrester DJ, Jacobson ER. Helminths of mariculture-reared green turtles (*Chelonia mydas mydas*) from Grand Cayman, British West Indies. Proc Helminthol Soc Wash 1980;47(1):142–4.

[38] Cordero T, Gardner ASC, Arellano-Blanco J, et al. Learedius learedi infection in black turtles (*Chelonia mydas agassizii*), Baja California Sur, Mexico. J Parasitol 2004;90(3):645–7.

[39] Frye F. Biomedical and surgical aspects of captive reptile husbandry. Malabar (FL): Krieger; 1991.

[40] Zwart P, Truyens E. Hexamitiasis in tortoises. Vet Parasitol 1975;1(2):175–83.

[41] Frank W, Bachmann U, Braun R. Aussergewöhnliche Todesfälle durch Amöbiasis bei einer Brückenechse (*Sphenodon punctatus*) bei jungen Suppenschildkröten (*Chelonia mydas*) und bei einer unechten Karettschildkröte (*Caretta caretta*) I. Amöbiasis bei *Sphenodon punctatus* [Unusual incidents of death caused by amoebiasis in a tuatara, (*Sphenodon punctatus*), young green turtles (*Chelonia mydas*) and a pseudo-loggerhead turtle (*Caretta caretta*) I. Amoebiasis in *Sphenodon punctatus*]. Salamandra (Frankf) 1976;12(2):94–102.

[42] Frank W, Sachsse W, Winkelsträter KH. Aussergewöhnliche Todesfälle durch Amöbiasis bei einer Brückenechse (*Sphenodon punctatus*) bei jungen Suppenschildkröten (*Chelonia mydas*) und bei einer unechten Karettschildkröte (*Caretta caretta*) II Amöbiasis bei *Chelonia mydas* und *Caretta caretta* [Unusual incidents of death caused by amoebiasis in a tuatara, (*Sphenodon punctatus*), young green turtles (*Chelonia mydas*) and a pseudo-loggerhead turtle (*Caretta caretta*). II. Amoebiasis in *Chelonia mydas* and *Caretta caretta*]. Salamandra (Frankf) 1976;12(2):120–6.

[43] Zwart P. Intraepithelial Protozoon, *Klossiella boae* n. sp. in the kidneys of a Boa constrictor. J Protozool 1964;11:261–3.

[44] Lainson R, Paperna I. *Tyzzeria boae* n. sp., (Apicomplexa: Eimeriidae), a new coccidium from the kidney of the snake boa constrictor (Serpentes: Boidae). Mem Inst Oswaldo Cruz 1994;89(4):523–30.

[45] Obwolo M, Zwart P. Prevalence of coccidiosis in reared Nile Crocodiles (*Crocodylus niloticus*) on a farm in Zimbabwe. The Zimbabwe Vet J 1992;23(2):73–8.

[46] Johnson CA. *Myxidium chelonarum* n. sp. (Cnidospora: Myxidiidae) from various North American turtles. Assoc SE Biol Bull 1969;16:56.

[47] Helke KL, Poynton SL. *Myxidium mackiei* (Myxosporea) in Indo-Gangetic flap-shelled turtles *Lissemys punctata andersonii*: parasite-host interaction and ultrastructure. Dis Aquat Org 2005;63:215–30.

[48] Jayasari M, Hoffman GL. Review of Myxidium (Protozoa: Myxozoa: Myxosporea). Protozool Abst 1982;6:61–91.

[49] Myxidium. Available at: http://www.afip.org/vetpath/WSC/wsc98/98wsc28.htm.

[50] Jacobson E-R, Green D-E, et al. Systemic microsporidiosis in inland bearded dragons (*Pogona vitticeps*). J Zoo Wildl Med 1998;29(3):315–23.

[51] Schumacher J, Jacobson ER, Homer BI, et al. Inclusion body disease in boid snakes. J Zoo Wildl Med 1994;24(4):511–24.

[52] Hauser B, Mettler F, Rübel A. Herpesvirus infection in two young boas. J Comp Pathol 1983;93:5515–9.

[53] Jacobson ER, Gaskin JM, Wahlquist H. Herpesvirus-like infection in map turtles. J Am Vet Med Assoc 1982;181:1322–4.

[54] Raidal SR, Ohara M, Hobbs RP, et al. Gram negative bacterial infections and cardiovascular parasitism in green sea turtles (*Chelonia mydas*). Aust Vet J 1998;76(6):415–7.

[55] Glazebrook JS, Campbell R. A survey of the diseases of marine turtles in northern Australian farmed turtles. Dis Aquat Org 1990;9(2):83–95.

[56] Wang W, Tu C, Hsy TY, et al. Fibrous, haemorrhagic and necrotic enteritis of soft-shell turtle (*Trionyx sinensis*). J Chinese Soc Vet Sci 1999;25(1):14–22.

[57] Frye FL, Corcoran JH. Spirochaetosis in an Asian box turtle, *Cuora flavomarginata*. In: Proceedings of the Fourth International Colloquium on Pathology and Therapy of Reptiles and Amphibians. Bad Nauheim, Germany: German Veterinary Association; 1991. p. 42–6.

[58] Abdulla PK, Karstad L. Experimental infections with *Leptospira pomona* in snakes and turtles. Zoonoses Res 1962;1:295–306.

[59] Zwart P, Cornelisse JL. Streptokokkensepsis mit Hautwucherungen bei Eidechsen [Sepsis due to streptococci, and proliferations of the skin]. Verhandl Ber 14 Int Symp Erkrk. Zoot Wroclaw, Poland; 1972. p. 265–9.

[60] McNamara TS, Gardiner C, Harris RK, et al. Streptococcal bacteriaemia in two Singapore house geckos (*Gekko monarchus*). J Zoo Wildl Dis 1994;25(1):161–6.

[61] Ippen R. Die spontane Tuberkulose bei Kaltblütern [Spontaneous tuberculosis in cold-blooded animals]. Nord Vet Med 1962;14(Suppl 1):184.

[62] Greer L, Strandberg JD, Whitaker BR. Mycobacterium chelonae osteoarthritis in a Kemp's Ridley sea turtle (*Lepidochelys kempii*). J Wildl Dis 2003;39(3):736–41.

[63] Brock JR, Nakamura RM, Miyahara AY, et al. Tuberculosis in Pacific green sea turtles, *Chelonia mydas*. Trans Am Fish Soc 1976;105(4):564–6.

[64] Oros J, Ramirez AS, Poveda JB, et al. Systemic mycosis caused by *Penicillium griseofulvum* in a Seychelles giant tortoise (*Megalochelys gigantea*). Vet Rec 1996;139(12):295–6.

[65] Ruiz JM, Arteaga E, Martinez J, et al. Cutaneous and renal geotrichosis in a giant tortoise (*Geochelone elephantophus*). Sabouraudia 1980;18:51–9.

[66] Manire C, Rhinehart HL, Sutton DA, et al. Disseminated mycotic infection caused by *Colletotrichum acutatum* in a Kemp's Ridley sea turtle (*Lepidochelys kempi*). J Clin Microbiol 2002;40(11):4273–80.

[67] Zarnik B. Untersuchungen über den Bau der Niere von Echidna und der Reptilienniere [Comparative studies on the structure of the kidney in Echidna and reptiles]. Jenaische Z f Naturwiss 1910;46:113–224.

[68] Cordier R. Études histophysiologiques sur le tube urinaire des reptiles [Histophysiologic studies on the urinary tube of reptiles]. Arch Biol (Liege) 1928;38:111–71.

[69] Spanner R. Bau und Kreislauf der Reptilienniere. I. Teil Blindschleichen [Structure and circulation of the reptilian kidney. Part 1. Slow worms]. Z f Anat Entw Gesch 1925;76: 64–90.

[70] Oros J, Tucker S, Fernández L, et al. Metastatic squamous cell carcinoma in two loggerhead sea turtles Caretta caretta. Dis Aquat Org 2004;58(2/3):245–50.

[71] Ippen R, Mladenov Z, Konstantinov A. Leukose mit elektronenoptischem Virusnachweis bei zwei Abgottschlangen (Boa constrictor) [Leucosis and electro-optical proof of a virus in two boas (Boa constrictor)]. Schweiz Arch Tierheilkd 1978;120:357–68.

[72] Oros J, Lorenzo H, Andrada M, et al. Type A-like retroviral particles in a metastatic intestinal adenocarcinoma in an emerald tree boa (Corallus caninus). Vet Pathol 2004;41(5): 515–8.

[73] Ippen R. Ein Beitrag zu Spontantumoren bei Reptilien [A contribution to spontaneous tumors in reptiles]. Verhdl Ber Int Symp Erkrkg Zoot 1972;14:409–18.

[74] Harshbarger J. Reptiles. In: Melby EC, Altman NH, editors. Handbook of laboratory animal science. Cleveland (OH): CRC Press; 1976. p. 343–56.

[75] Harshbarger J. Activities reports registry of tumors in lower animals, 1965–1973. Washington, DC: Smithsonian Institute Press; 1974. p. 80.

[76] Frye FL, Barten SI. Myelogenous leukaemia in a helmeted turtle, Pelomedusa subrufa. Verhdl Ber Int Symp Erkrkg Zoot 1991;33:412–3.

[77] Harshbarger J. Activities reports registry of tumors in lower animals, 1977 supplement. Washington, DC: Smithsonian Institute Press; 1978. p. 44.

[78] Norton TM, Jacobson ER, Sundberg JP. Cutaneous fibropapillomas and renal myxofibroma in a green turtle, Chelonia mydas. J Wildl Dis 1990;26(2):265–70.

[79] Oros J, Torrent A, Espinosa de los Monteros A. Multicentric lymphoblastic lymphoma in a loggerhead sea turtle (Caretta caretta). Vet Pathol 2001;38(4):464–7.

[80] Martin JC, Schelling SH, Pokras MA. Gastric adenocarcinoma in a Florida indigo snake (Drymarchon corais couperi). J Zoo Wildl Med 1994;25(1):133–7.

[81] Barten SL, Davis K, Harris RK, et al. Renal cell carcinoma with metastases in a corn snake (Elaphe guttata). J Zoo Wildl Med 1994;25(1):123–7.

[82] Voprsalek T, Simunek J. Vitamin A deficiency in tortoises. Tieraerztl Umsch 1996;51(11): 711.

[83] Elkan E, Zwart P. The ocular disease of young terrapins caused by vitamin A deficiency. Pathol Vet 1967;4:201–22.

[84] Ippen R, Konstantinov A. Durch Vitamin-A-Mangel bedingte Nierenveränderungen bei einem Ganges-Gavial (Gavialis gangeticus) [Renal changes in gharial (Gavialis gangeticus) due to vitamin A deficiency]. Verh Ber Erkrg Zootiere 1981;23:127–31.

[85] Golob Z, Kobal S. Example of reptile poisoning by azinphos-methyl and its determination in biological extracts by thin layer chromatography. Herpetopathologia. In: Proceedings of the Fifth International Symposium on Pathology of Reptiles and Amphibians. Alphen aan den Rijn, The Netherlands: 1995. 31–3-02–04: p. 317–20.

[86] Zwart P, Teunis SFM, Cornelissen JMM. Monocercomoniasis in reptiles. Journal of Zoo Animal Medicine 1984;15:129–34.

[87] Frank W. Endoparasites. In: Cooper JE, Jackson OF, editors. Diseases of the reptilian, vol. 1. London: Academic Press; 1981. p. 295–9.

[88] Innis CJ, Kincaid AL. Bilateral calcium phosphate ureteroliths and Spirorchid trematode infection in a red-eared slider turtle, Trachemys scripta elegans, with a review of the pathology of spirorchiasis. Bulletin of the Association of Reptilian and Amphibian Veterinarians 1999; 9(30):32–5.

[89] Morrissey M. Urolithiasis in a green iguana. Exotic Pet Practice 1999;4(7):53.

[90] An M, Jang I. A case report: Iguana iguana with cystic calculus. Korean Journal of Veterinary Clinical Medicine 1998;15(2):472–5.

[91] Virchow R. Ein grosser Blasen-(Cloaken?-)Stein von einer Meeresschildkröte [A large urinary (cloacal?-) calculus in a sea turtle]. Virchows Arch 1878;73:629–30.

[92] Mebs D. Harnsteine bei Schildkröten [Urinary stones in chelonians]. Salamandra (Frankf) 1965;1:47–9.

[93] Homer B, Berry KH, Brown MB. Pathology of diseases in wild desert tortoises from California. J Wildl Dis 1998;34(3):508–23.

[94] Henke S, Pence DB, Tran RM. Urinary bladders of freshwater turtles as a renal physiology model potentially biased by monogenean infections. Lab Anim Sci 1990;40(2):172–7.

ELSEVIER
SAUNDERS

VETERINARY
CLINICS
Exotic Animal Practice

Vet Clin Exot Anim 9 (2006) 161–174

Renal Diseases of Reptiles

Paolo Selleri, Dr Med Vet, PhD[a,b,*],
Stephen J. Hernandez-Divers, BVM, DZoomed,
MRCVS, DACZM, RCVS[c]

[a]Centro Veterinario Specialistico—Animali Esotici, Via Sandro Giovannini, 51/53,
00179 Rome, Italy
[b]Dipartimento di Scienze Cliniche Veterinarie, Facoltà di Medicina Veterinaria,
viale dell' Università 16, 35020 Legnaro, Padua, Italy
[c]Department of Small Animal Medicine and Surgery, College of Veterinary Medicine,
University of Georgia, Athens, GA 30602, USA

Practicing exotic species medicine requires a broad depth of knowledge, including knowledge of diseases without pathognomonic clinical signs. In most cases, signs of disease are not obvious until the animal is severely compromised. Knowledge of biologic peculiarities and environmental requirements are indispensable when dealing with exotic species (Figs. 1 and 2). Renal disease is one of the most common problems in reptilian medicine. Herbivorous species seem to be more susceptible than carnivores. The causation may be multifactorial, and the signs are often nonspecific. Prevention is preferred to treatment, and a comprehensive health program, which includes quarantine, routine health screens during annual examinations, and necropsy examinations of all animals that die is desirable.

Clinical investigation

A detailed history is crucial to understand if a reptile may be at risk of metabolic disorders (eg, diet with a poor calcium to phosphorus ratio [Ca:P], lack of broad-spectrum lighting) or immunocompromised (eg, chronic low temperature, presence of a dominating male in the same enclosure) and thus prone to infectious diseases. A significant portion of the examination of a reptile with renal failure must be dedicated to understanding how the animal has been fed and kept in captivity. It is also important to consider the past history of the reptile that may suggest the cause of the

---

* Corresponding author. Via Ambrogio Fusinieri, 50, 00149 Rome, Italy.
  E-mail address: pseller@tin.it (P. Selleri).

vetexotic.theclinics.com

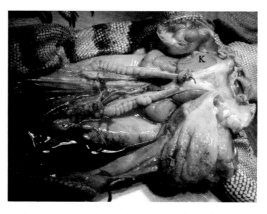

Fig. 1. Necropsy of a female iguana (*Iguana iguana*) showing enlarged kidneys. The intestinal tract has been removed. K, kidney; O, ovary.

current illness (eg, animals with secondary hyperparathyroidism may develop renal insufficiency because of the cytotoxic effects of excess of parathyroid hormone [1]).

Physical investigation

Reptiles in advanced renal failure often show obvious symptoms, but it may be difficult to detect clinical signs in the early stages of the disease. Thus, the examination must be meticulous. Core body temperature of ectothermic animals is an important parameter and is collected rectally during the examination with a thermometer capable of a wide range. Internal temperatures lower than the preferred body temperature may suggest that the animal is ill or is maintained in suboptimal conditions. When interpreting

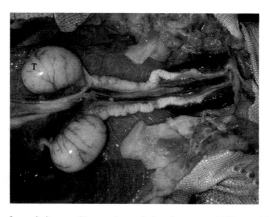

Fig. 2. Necropsy of a male iguana (*Iguana iguana*) showing normal kidneys. The intestinal tract has been removed. K, kidney; T, testis.

the reptile's temperature reading, consider the immediate environmental conditions and time away from the animal's captive habitat.

Body weight should always be assessed [2]; changes are uncommon in acute renal failure, whereas chronic renal disease can lead to weight loss and dehydration. Dehydration may be inferred from reductions in skin elasticity, saliva, and ocular secretions [3].

Animals with severe renal impairment will present with weakness, depression, and myoclonus. Diseases that result in increased urinary or intestinal loss of albumin may result in hypoalbuminemia and edema [4].

In snakes the kidneys are not easy to locate but may be palpated when enlarged. In chelonians, because of the protective carapace, the retrocoelomic position of the kidneys makes them nonpalpable. In lizards, enlarged kidneys may be palpated in the caudal to mid-coelom, sometimes just cranial to the pelvis, depending on the species. In iguanids, cloacal palpation may help evaluate the size of the intrapelvic kidneys (Fig. 3).

Clinicopathology

Blood collection

In lizards, blood is most commonly collected from the ventral caudal (tail) vein. The ventral abdominal vein can also be used and may be preferred in those lizards prone to tail autotomy. The jugular vein is also available but is more complicated to access.

In snakes, blood collection from the ventral caudal (tail) vein and cardiocentesis are the most practical means.

In chelonians, blood may be collected from many sites, but the first choice should be the jugular vein. Even if the procedure seems more complicated than using other sites, lymph contamination is less likely, and the sample is more reliable.

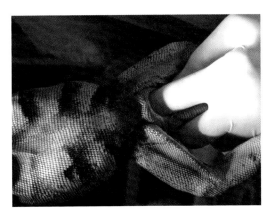

Fig. 3. Transcloacal palpation of the kidneys in an iguana (*Iguana iguana*).

Blood that contains no anticoagulant provides the best sample for evaluating blood films; therefore a blood film should be made immediately after collection. Lithium heparin has been considered the best anticoagulant in reptile hematology and biochemistry. Recently, ethylenediaminetetraacetic acid (EDTA) has been shown to be preferable for some squamates [5].

Hematology

Other than species, several other factors such as sex, age, and season may influence hematologic parameters [6]. Pathologic elevations of the packed cell volume are usually related to dehydration [3]. In chronic cases, a nonregenerative anemia may also be present. When both anemia and dehydration exist, the packed cell volume could be normal and mask hemoconcentration. In acute cases, the reptile's white blood cell count may be elevated, usually because of heterophilia. Leukocyte changes are less common in chronic cases, but mild leukocytosis and monocytosis may be found. Eosinophilia may be expected when the kidneys are affected by parasitic diseases such as trematodiasis in boa constrictors and hexamitiasis of certain chelonians.

When reptiles are constantly exposed to temperatures lower than their preferred body temperature zone, they may become immunocompromised and fail to demonstrate an appropriated leukocyte response, even in the face of overwhelming infection.

Biochemistry

Renal function in reptiles cannot be evaluated by blood biochemistry tests alone, but several parameters may be useful in the assessment of renal disease.

Uric acid is the final product of nitrogenous metabolism in most reptiles. A reduction of the renal secretion of uric acid leads to hyperuricemia, a condition that can also be caused by profound dehydration and reduction in renal blood flow. In desert species and in postprandial samples from carnivorous reptiles, uric acid values may be physiologically elevated [6]. In cases of chronic renal disease, significant elevations of uric acid are usually apparent only when profound renal damage has occurred [6].

In end-stage renal disease, blood uric acid levels rise above 24.5 mg/dL (1457 µmol/L) and give rise to visceral and articular gout (Fig. 4) [7,8].

Production and excretion of urea are variable in most reptiles. In aquatic chelonians, however, urea excretion is a consistent fraction of nitrogen excretion, and urea may be of clinical value [9]. Unless it is clearly outside the reference range, a single urea result is of limited value because of inter- and intraspecies variability. Serial samples are more informative and may aid in the assessment of dehydration, renal dysfunction, and response to therapy [10].

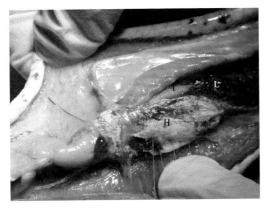

Fig. 4. Uric acid deposition in the pericardial sac of a Savu python (*Liasis savuensis*). H, heart; L, lung; T, trachea.

Creatinine assays are highly variable and are not reliable because their results are elevated only after severe renal compromise has occurred [11].

Aspartate aminotransferase, creatinine phosphokinase, and lactate dehydrogenase levels may also be elevated during acute renal disease, but their wide tissue abundance makes them a nonspecific marker of renal disease [12]. Because of the presence of aspartate aminotransferase in the epithelial cells of the proximal tubule, any lesion occurring there results in a dramatic elevation of aspartate aminotransferase [13].

γ-Glutamyl transferase is an enzyme present in the brush border of the renal tubule. Further investigations are required to consider γ-glutamyl transferase a reliable urinary marker of renal tubular disease. Chronic glomerular disease can cause a loss of low molecular weight proteins leading to hypoalbuminemia and, consequently, edema. Edema may be present when glomerular damage causes profound renal insufficiency [4].

One of the most important indicators of iguanid renal function is the Ca:P ratio. This parameter may be influenced by several factors that must be kept in mind when diagnosing renal disorders. The optimal Ca:P ratio for most vertebrates lies within a range of 1.5:1 to 2:1 [14]. In cases of reptilian renal disease, often the first plasma biochemical indicator is the reduction of this ratio; however, an altered Ca:P ratio can also occur late in course of disease.

When evaluating the Ca:P ratio, the clinician must not forget that assessing the calcium value is problematic because it may be affected by many factors. Most automated analyzers measure total serum calcium concentration, which consists of biologically active, ionized calcium (50%), protein-bound calcium (40%), and calcium complexes (10%). Because of extensive protein binding, total serum calcium concentration is decreased by hypoalbuminemia [15]. Measurement of ionized calcium might be more appropriate in assessing the physiologic status of the reptile patient [16,17]. The biologically active, ionized fraction of calcium can be determined directly. Special sample handling, use of specialized instrumentation, and adjustments for sample pH are necessary to ensure accuracy in measuring serum concentration of ionized calcium.

The Ca:P ratio may also be affected by gender and reproductive status. Ovulating females have high circulating egg proteins and often exhibit physiologically normal elevation of calcium up to 24 mg/dL.

Although not validated in reptiles, useful information may be obtained calculating the solubility index (multiplying calcium × phosphorous), which may help determine the therapeutic needs for calcium, phosphorus restriction or phosphorus binders, diuresis, and vitamin D_3 [6,18]. In mammals, the normal index value is less than 9 (in mmol/L) or 55 (in mg/dL). When the solubility index increases to values between 9 and 12 (55–70 mg/dL), mineralization of diseased tissue can occur. When values are over 12 (>70 mg/dL), metastatic mineralization of healthy tissue can take place.

Sodium, potassium, and chloride can show shifts from normal values. Hyponatremia and hyperkalemia may be expected from dysfunction of the distal tubules, cloaca, colon, or bladder [6], but more detailed evaluation is required of both healthy and renal-diseased animals.

Renal function testing

Plasma elevations of nitrogenous metabolites are not reliable indicators of renal function because they can be affected by hydration status, and pathologic changes tend to occur late in the course of disease. Scintigraphy, CT, and MRI have been used to measure renal blood flow or renal clearance of radioactive nuclides or contrast agents [19–21]. Other techniques rely on determining the plasma clearance of an exogenous compound (eg, phenosulfonphthalein, inulin, creatinine); these techniques require intravenous drug administration, serial blood sampling, and catheterization for urine collection. Because of the postrenal modification of urine in the reptilian cloaca, colon, or bladder, it is essential to catheterize the ureters to differentiate the roles of glomerular filtration and tubular transport from those of the cloaca, colon, and bladder [9].

Iohexol clearance studies have proven to be a safe and effective method for estimating glomerular filtration rate and renal function. A recent study validated this methodology in reptiles [22]. Iohexol is a non-ionic radiographic iodine contrast medium of low osmolarity. It is excreted exclusively by glomerular filtration with negligible extrarenal elimination in mammals [23]. The plasma clearance of iohexol can be determined by analysis of plasma iohexol concentration over time after a single intravenous injection. This method has the distinct advantage of relying on blood collection and not urinary catheterization for the collection of urine; furthermore it does not require expensive equipment to be performed. The green iguana needs to be fasted and hydrated for 24 hours before the iohexol is administered. The recommended dose for the green iguana is 75 mg/kg intravenously. To reduce the risk of perivascular injection, intravenous catheterization is recommended. Blood samples are collected 4, 8, and 24 hours after the injection and can be sent on ice for iohexol assays and glomerular filtration rate calculation to the Diagnostic Center for Population and Animal Health (Michigan State University, East Lansing, Michigan 48824).

Urinalysis

Urinalysis is not as clinically useful in reptile medicine as in mammalian medicine. The intimate anatomic relationship between the urinary system and the digestive tract makes reptile urine potentially not sterile. The lack of a loop of Henle makes the kidney unable to produce hypertonic urine. Finally, postrenal modifications of urine occur in the reptilian cloaca, colon, or bladder, potentially changing the composition of ureteral urine. For research purposes it is essential to catheterize the ureters to differentiate the roles of glomerular filtration and tubular transport from those of the cloaca, colon, and bladder [9]. Despite all these limitations, urine samples may still be submitted for cytology to detect inflammation, infection, renal casts, and parasites.

Diagnostic imaging techniques

Radiography

Several primary and secondary signs of renal disease may be identified using radiology. In iguanids (*Iguana* spp), the normal kidneys are located in the pelvic canal and cannot be appreciated on radiographs. Dorsoventral and lateral radiographs, however, are useful for assessing renomegaly [24] and the presence of uroliths and macroscopic soft tissue mineralization. The urinary bladder is not a distinct radiographic structure in iguanid lizards [25].

In chelonians, the kidneys are located in the dorsocaudal region and are impossible to identify when normal [26]. Radiology may identify secondary signs of renal disease.

In lizards, enlarged kidneys may reduce the volume of the pelvic canal causing extramural obstruction of the colon and subsequent constipation. Obstructive dystocia can also be the result of renal enlargement.

When the plain radiograph indicate a mass in the dorsocaudal part of the coelom, contrast studies (eg, intracoelomic injection of air, gastrointestinal barium) can be used to help differentiate the kidney from other soft tissues structures [3]. Intravenous urography can be applied to evaluate the kidneys and the ureters better. An intravenous catheter is placed in the right jugular vein, 800–1000 mg/kg of aqueous iodine contrast media (iopamidole) is injected, and serial dorsoventral and lateral radiographs are taken at 0, 0.5, 2, 5, 15, 30, and 60 minutes [3]. When renal disease leads to secondary hyperparathyroidism, radiographs may show an overall decrease in bone density. Conventional radiography requires 40% loss of mineralization before changes in bone opacity can be detected [27]. Dual-energy x-ray absorptiometry is the technique of choice for measuring bone density in iguanas [28].

Ultrasonography

Ultrasonography is a noninvasive technique to evaluate renal parenchyma dimensions and structure. For best results, a probe with a frequency of 7.5 to 10 mHz is recommended, particularly when dealing with small animals. When dealing with ectothermic animals, it is important not to expose the animal to rapid temperature changes. Because ultrasonography can last several minutes, it is wise to warm the gel. To limit the heat loss, ultrasonography can be performed by placing the reptile in a tank of warm water and using a probe with a waterproof protective device. This procedure is an excellent technique to enhance the quality of the image, especially in snakes. Water is the best medium for conducting ultrasound, because it easily enters the interscale space, offering the best ultrasound image. The animal is placed in ventral recumbency. Manual restraint is usually adequate.

In chelonians, ultrasonography is is particularly useful because coelomic palpation is difficult. When examining powerful animals, sedation is advised to avoid damage to the transducer when it is trapped between the shell and the hind limb. The legs are extended caudally, and the transducer is inserted in the prefemoral acoustic window. Because of the limited dimensions of the prefemoral fossa, a sector probe should be used. The thin-walled bladder may contain a large amount of fluid. When full, the urinary bladder may expand, filling the coelomic cavity and making it difficult to distinguish urine from coelomic effusion. Hyperechoic urate crystals and calculi generate a shadow. Moving the chelonian while performing ultrasonography helps with differentiation [26]. The chelonian kidney is inspected by directing the probe dorsally. The medulla often appears hypoechoic and triangular-oval in shape. Ultrasonography allows the visualization of urate deposition, mineralization, and neoplasia.

In iguanids the bony pelvis obstructs ultrasonic waves, and therefore the transducer must be placed cranial to the hind limb and angled caudally toward the center of the pelvic canal (Fig. 5). The caudal pole of the kidney can be inspected by placing the transducer ventrally to the lateral processes of the vertebrae and caudal to the pelvic bone. The normal renal parenchyma is uniform, because no cortex and medulla are distinguishable.

In snakes, ultrasonography is useful for the evaluation of renal enlargement, mineralization, and neoplasia.

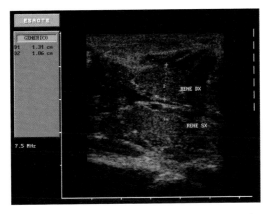

Fig. 5. Ultrasonography of the cranial pole of the enlarged kidneys of a female iguana (*Iguana iguana*). The transducer is placed cranial to the hindlimb.

Scintigraphy

Experimental studies at the University of Tennessee indicate that the kidney of green iguanas can be evaluated scintigraphically by the use of technetium dimercaptosuccinic acid. This technique may be potentially useful for diagnosis of renal failure [19].

Endoscopy

In reptilian medicine, endoscopy is an important diagnostic tool for the evaluation of renal disease. The results of clinicopathological tests on blood specimens are often inconclusive, and the diagnosis often is centered on visualization of the affected organ to evaluate its external surface, borders, and colors. Endoscopy is rapid to perform, so anesthesia can be brief.

Small (2.7-mm), rigid endoscopes are commonly available to the exotic practitioner. Their size and ability to accommodate various instruments makes endoscopy indispensable for diagnosis, therapy, and surgery.

To perform a coelioscopy in lizards, the anesthetized animal is placed in lateral recumbency, ventilated, and prepared for aseptic surgery. In iguanas, the skin is incised at a paralumbar site. In most cases, a left lateral approach is preferred because it allows a rapid visualization of other organs as well. If the animal's condition permits, endoscopy should be performed after a 2-day fast to simplify the examination. The kidneys in the pelvic canal are difficult to reach because of fat bodies, the urinary bladder, and the distal tract of the colon. Coelomic cavity insufflation with CO_2 is routine.

In chelonians, the kidneys can be reached by transcoelomic or extracoelomic approaches. For the transcoelomic approach, the coelomic cavity is entered by making an incision followed by blunt entry into the coelom using hemostats. With the extracoelomic approach the endoscope does not enter the coelomic cavity. The use of the protection sheath is mandatory when performing this technique. Once the tip of the endoscope has passed the skin incision, it is oriented in a caudodorsal direction and moved forward between the coelomic aponeurosis and the iliacus muscle. Insufflation and lateral movements of the sheathed endoscope help the advancement under direct visual control and the identification of the caudal aspect of the kidney [10].

Anatomic features of snakes limit coelioscopy. The elongated shape of ophidians requires several entries to perform a complete survey. Endoscopy can also be complicated by diffuse fat located in the caudal part of the coelomic cavity and difficult insufflation.

Renal biopsy

Histologic examination of the renal parenchyma plays a fundamental role in the diagnosis of renal disease. Diseased renal parenchyma has poor regenerative capacity; therefore kidney biopsy is an important step in the early diagnostic process [18].

In iguanas, the caudal pole of the kidney extends caudally to the pelvic bones, and the biopsy can be collected using a caudal tail cut-down technique. A cutaneous incision is made parallel to the long axis of the tail, with a maximal length of 3 to 4 cm, beginning a few millimeters beyond the angle of the hind limb and the tail. The caudal-most part of the kidneys is reached by blunt dissection through the coccygeal muscles. This technique is useful when the kidneys are not very enlarged or are affected by diffuse diseases or if celiotomy is contraindicated. If bleeding should arise from the biopsy site, it can be easily controlled by pressure or cauterization with radiosurgery.

When kidneys are significantly enlarged, celiotomy allows a direct inspection and sampling from both organs. The kidney can be approached using a standard paramedian technique. In obvious renomegaly it may be sufficient to incise the skin directly over the swelling [29].

An ultrasound-guided biopsy can be performed in many reptiles. This technique requires a skilled operator and high-quality equipment. This technique permits an evaluation of tissue homogeneity and helps localize the lesions, allowing the clinician to sample the affected areas while avoiding other organs. Ultrasound-guided biopsy is used in large animals and when the kidneys are enlarged and easily identified. Some biopsies are not easy to perform because of the risk of damaging other thin-walled structures such as the urinary bladder, which may often be difficult to identify.

Endoscopic renal biopsy is a common technique. Once the kidney is visualized, to avoid crushing the histologic specimen, it is better to incise the coelomic and renal membranes with endoscopic scissors and expose the kidney before collecting the biopsy. To obtain a renal biopsy in a snake, insert the rigid endoscope through an incision made in the last caudal fourth of the coelomic cavity at the second row of lateral scales, as for standard celiotomy, but limit the length of the incision to 2 to 4 mm [30].

Therapy

The first goal of the therapy is to stabilize the critical patient. The first steps must be directed to bringing the reptile into its optimal range of temperature. It is essential to determine the animal's body weight and its hydration status by evaluating packed cell volume and total protein. Once the cause of the disease is identified, more specific therapy can support remaining renal function. It is essential to correct dehydration, restore urine excretion, and adjust electrolytic and acid-base imbalances. Euthanasia must be considered in terminal cases [31].

Ensuring proper hydration is one of the most important aspects of managing renal disease in reptiles. Fluids should always be warmed to help raise the animal's temperature to the preferred body temperature. The oral route is less painful for the animal and should be preferred when possible.

The parenteral routes for fluid therapy include intracoelomic, intravenous, or intraosseous routes. Large amounts of fluids should not be administered subcutaneously, especially when dealing with reptiles with little subcutaneous space, such as snakes. To perform intraosseous catheterization, a spinal needle is inserted distally through the tibial crest and into the medullary cavity. After the stylet is removed, the needle is connected to an infusion pump. Fluids are infused at a rate of about 1 mL/kg/h. In critical cases, fluids may be infused at up to 5 mL/kg/h for the first 3 hours. Expansion of circulating volume improves renal blood flow and function, promoting the correction of acid–base and electrolytic imbalances. For chronically dehydrated patients, care is required to avoid iatrogenic hypoalbuminemia and rapid dilution of plasma electrolytes. In these cases a reduction of parenteral fluid therapy is advised [18].

Reptiles have more body water (63%–74% by weight) [32] than mammals (60% by weight) [33]. The fluid amount in the intracellular space (45.8%–58.0%) [32] is also higher than in mammals (40%) [33]. Conversely, reptiles have lower volumes of interstitial, plasma, and extracellular fluids [32]. For this reason, severe dehydration is best treated by using hypotonic fluids to reduce the osmolality of extracellular fluids and to promote the shift of water into the intracellular space [34].

In clinical practice, 25 to 35 mL/kg of a mixed solution of 0.18% NaCl and 4% dextrose or half-strength lactated Ringer's solution with 2% to 5% dextrose should be given in the intracoelomic cavity over 24 hours [35]. When hyperkalemia is present, lactated Ringer's solution may be contraindicated because of its potassium content.

In animals with anuria, administer diuretics (Table 1) such as mannitol 20% (2 mL/kg intravenously in 24 hours) or furosemide (2–5 mg/kg intravenously or intramuscularly in 24 hours). Once the acute crisis is over, fluid administration may be continued in other ways: through high humidity by nebulization, soaking food in water, using water drip-dispensers, and providing bathing facilities.

Table 1
Medications commonly used in reptiles with renal diseases

Agent	Dose	Comments
Mannitol 20%	2 mL/kg IV over 24 h	Diuretic
Furosemide	2–5 mg/kg IM in 24 h	Diuretic
Allopurinol	20 mg/kg PO q 24 h	Decreases uric acid formation
Probenecid	2–4 mg/kg PO SID	Increases uric acid excretion
Sulphapirazole	1–3 mg/kg PO SID	Increases uric acid excretion
Calcium gluconate	50–100 mg/kg IM q 6 h	Seizures or flaccid paresis
Calcium gluconate	400 mg/kg IV over 24 h	Seizures or flaccid paresis
Aluminum hydroxide	15–45 mg/kg PO SID	Decreases intestinal absorption of phosphorus
Calcium carbonate	250 mg/kg PO SID	Decreases intestinal absorption of phosphorus
Ca-EDTA	20 mg/kg IM, IV q 24 h	Calcium chelating agent
Stanozolole	5 mg/kg IM q 7 d	Stimulates appetite
Enrofloxacin	5–10 mg/kg PO, IM, SC SID	
Metronidazole	20 mg/kg q 48 h	Very effective against anaerobes

Significant increases of uric acid concentrations above normal may indicate severe renal damage. If serum uric acid is over 1457 μmol/L (24.5 mg/dL), gout (deposition of uric acid crystals in tissues) may develop. Allopurinol (20 mg/kg by mouth once a day) may decrease the hepatic production of uric acid. Probenecid (2–4 mg/kg by mouth once a day) and sulphapyrazole (1–3 mg/kg by mouth once a day) may prevent tubular reabsorbtion of uric acid and theoretically increase its excretion.

Hypocalcemia is a common anomaly found in renal failure and may lead to tetany, seizures, and death. Clinical signs often improve rapidly within 48 hours of starting calcium-gluconate administration (100 mg/kg intramuscularly every 6 hours or 400 mg/kg intravenously given over a 24-hour period) and phosphorus-chelating agents. Blood calcium levels must be evaluated frequently during the following days to weeks, with dosages adjusted accordingly. After the acute phase is over, calcium administration may be continued orally.

Substances containing vitamin D_3 are generally avoided because they can cause iatrogenic hypercalcemia and tissue calcification. In human medicine, however, cholecalciferol is used as a closely titrated treatment for secondary renal hyperparathyroidism. Exposure to unfiltered UV light allows correct production of vitamin D_3 (assuming that hydroxycholecalciferol hydroxylation to 1.25-dihydroxycholecalciferol is not compromised by renal damage). Hypercalcemia caused by vitamin D_3 toxicosis may induce renal tubule dysfunction because of cellular necrosis. In these cases it is obviously necessary to stop vitamin D_3 administration and consider the use of calcium-chelating agents such as calcium disodium ethylene diamine tetracetate (Ca-EDTA) at 20 mg/kg intramuscularly or intravenously every 24 hours or aluminum hydroxyde at 15 to 45 mg/kg orally twice a day.

Hyperphosphatemia can often be pronounced in cases of renal diseases. In the initial stages diuresis helps reduce plasma phosphorus. Enteric phosphorus-chelating agents such as aluminum hydroxide (15–45 mg/kg orally twice a day) or calcium carbonate (250 mg/kg orally twice a day) may be used for long-term management.

When renal disease results from infectious causes, it is essential to biopsy the kidney for histopathologic evaluation, culture, and antibacterial sensitivity testing to direct appropriate therapy.

Anabolic hormones such as stanozolol (5 mg/kg intramuscularly every 7 days) can be used to stimulate appetite and reduce protein catabolism and purine degradation [36]. Even if not present in reptiles, these hormones are expected to have the positive effect of stimulating erythropoiesis and cellular metabolism.

When they impair renal function, ureteral or renal uroliths must be removed surgically. Because of the location of the kidneys, surgical ureterolith removal may be difficult and require a partial nephrectomy or unilateral nephrectomy.

References

[1] Massry SG, Fadda GZ. Chronic renal failure is a state of cellular calcium toxicity. Am J Kidney Dis 1993;21:81–6.

[2] Divers SJ. Clinical evaluation of reptiles. Vet Clin North Am Exotic Anim Pract 1999;2(2): 291–331.

[3] Hernandez-Divers SJ. Green Iguana nephrology. A review of diagnostic techniques. Vet Clin North Am Exotic Anim Pract 2003;6:233–50.

[4] Miller HA. Urinary diseases of reptiles: pathophysiology and diagnosis. Seminars in Avian and Exotic Pet Medicine 1998;7(2):93–103.

[5] Hanley CS, Hernandez-Divers SJ, Bush S, et al. Comparison of the effect of dipotassium ethylenediaminetetraacetic acid and lithium heparin on hematologic values in the green iguana (Iguana iguana). J Zoo Wildl Med 2004;35(3):328–32.

[6] Divers SJ. Reptilian renal and reproductive disease diagnosis. In: Fudge AM, editor. Laboratory medicine. Avian and exotic pets. Philadelphia: W.B. Saunders; 2000. p. 217–22.

[7] Minnich JE. The use of water. In: Gans C, Harvey Pough F, editors. Biology of the Reptilia, vol. 12, Physiological ecology. London: Academic Press; 1982. p. 325–95.

[8] Zwart P. Urogenital system. In: Beynon PH, editor. Manual of reptiles. Cheltenham (UK): British Small Animal Veterinary Association; 1992. p. 117–27.

[9] Dantzler WH. Renal function (with special emphasis on nitrogen excretion). In: Gans C, Dawson WR, editors. Biology of the Reptilia,vol. 5, Physiology A. London: Academic Press; 1976. p. 447–503.

[10] Hernandez-Divers SJ. Endoscopic renal evaluation and biopsy in chelonia. Vet Rec 2004; 154(3):73–80.

[11] Boyer TH. Clinicopathologic findings of twelve case of renal failure in Iguana iguana. In: Proceedings of the Second Annual Conference of the Association of Reptilian and Amphibian Veterinarians. Tampa (FL): Association of Reptilian and Amphibian Veterinarians; 1995. p. 113.

[12] Wagner RA, Wetzel R. Tissue and plasma enzyme activities in juvenile green iguanas. Am J Vet Res 1999;60(2):201–3.

[13] Suedmeyer K. Hypocalcemia and hyperphosphatemia in a Green Iguana with concurrent elevation of serum glutamic oxalic transaminase. Bulletin of the Association of Reptilian and Amphibian Veterinarians 1995;5(3):5–6.

[14] Fowler ME. Metabolic bone disease. In: Fowler ME, editor. Zoo and wild animal medicine. 2nd edition. Philadelphia: W.B. Saunders; 1986. p. 70–90.

[15] Nelson RW, Turnwald GH, Willard MD. Endocrine metabolic and lipid disorders. In: Willard MD, Tvedten H, Turnwald GH, editors. Small animal diagnosis by laboratory methods. 3rd edition. Philadelphia: W.B. Saunders; 1999. p. 136–71.

[16] Mader DR. Reptilian metabolic disorders. In: Fudge AM, editor. Laboratory medicine. Avian and exotic pets. Philadelphia: W.B. Saunders; 2000. p. 210–6.

[17] Dennis PM, Bennett RA, Harr KE, et al. Plasma concentration of ionized calcium in healthy iguanas. J Am Vet Med Assoc 2001;219(3):326–8.

[18] Divers SJ. Clinician's approach to renal disease in lizards. In: Proceedings of the Fourth Annual Conference of the ARAV. Houston (TX): Association of Reptilian and Amphibian Veterinarians; 1997. p. 5–11.

[19] Greer LL, Daniel GB, Shearn-Bochsler VI, et al. Evaluation of the use of technetium Tc 99m diethylenetriamine pentaacetic acid and technetium Tc 99m dimercaptosuccinic acid for scintigraphy imaging of the kidneys in green iguanas (*Iguana iguana*). Am J Vet Res 2005; 66:87–92.

[20] Gumpemberg M. Computed tomography. In: McArthur S, editor. Medicine and surgery of tortoises and turtles. Oxford, UK: Blackwell Publishing; 2004. p. 235–8.

[21] Calvert I. Magnetic resonance imaging. In: McArthur S, editor. Medicine and surgery of tortoises and turtles. Blackwell Publishing; 2004. p. 227–35.

[22] Hernandez-Divers SJ. Renal evaluation in the Green Iguana *(Iguana iguana)*: assessment of plasma biochemistry, glomerular filtration rate, and endoscopic biopsy. J Zoo Wildl Med 2005;36:155–68.

[23] Nilsson-Ehle P, Grubb A. New markers for the determination of GFR: iohexol clearance and cystatin C serum concentration. Kidney Int Suppl 1994;47:17–9.

[24] Hernandez-Divers SM, Hernandez-Divers SJ. Diagnostic imaging of reptiles. In Pract 2001; 23(7):170–86.

[25] Newel SM. Diagnostic imaging. In: Jacobson ER, editor. Biology, husbandry and medicine of the Green Iguana. Malabar (FL): Krieger Publishing; 2003. p. 168–77.

[26] Wilkinson R, Hernandez-Divers SJ, LaFortune M, et al. Diagnostic imaging techniques. In: McArthur S, editor. Medicine and surgery of tortoises and turtles. Oxford, UK: Blackwell Publishing; 2004. p. 187–238.

[27] Lauten SD. Use of dual energy X-ray absorptiometry for non invasive body composition measurements in clinically normal dogs. Am J Vet Res 2001;62:1295–301.

[28] Grier SJ. The use of dual-energy X-ray absorptiometry in animals. Invest Radiol 1996;31: 50–62.

[29] Frye FL. Percutaneous hepatic and renal biopsy employing the anchor soft tissue biopsy device. In: Proceedings of the North American Veterinary Conference, vol . 11. Orlando (FL): North American Veterinary Conference; 1997. p. 732.

[30] Hernandez-Divers SJ. Diagnostic and surgical endoscopy. Basic exotic animal endoscopy course. Athens (GA): University of Georgia; 2004.

[31] Waters M. A guide to lizards [CD-rom]. Hatfield, Herts, UK: Royal Veterinary College; 1999.

[32] Thorson TB. Body fluid partitioning in the Reptilia. Copeia 1968;3:592.

[33] Facello C. Il sangue. In: Fisiologia degli animali domestici con elementi di etologia. Bologna, Italy: UTET; 1992. p. 309–50.

[34] Shumacher J. Fluid therapy in reptiles. In: Bonagura JD. Kirk's current veterinary therapy XIII. Philadelphia: WB Saunders; 1999. p. 1170–4.

[35] Jarchow JL. Hospital care of the reptile patient. In: Thurmon JC, editor. Exotic animals. New York: Churchill Livingstone; 1988. p. 19.

[36] Gauvin J. Drug therapy in reptiles. Seminars in Avian and Exotic Pet Medicine 1993;2: 48–59.

ELSEVIER
SAUNDERS

VETERINARY
CLINICS
Exotic Animal Practice

Vet Clin Exot Anim 9 (2006) 175–188

Amphibian Renal Disease

Todd R. Cecil, DVM

*Avian and Exotic Animal Hospital, 2317 Hotel Circle South, Suite C,
San Diego, CA 92108, USA*

Amphibians by nature have an intimate connection with the aquatic environment at some stage of development and fight an osmotic battle due to the influx of water. Many amphibians have acquired a more terrestrial existence at later stages of development and consequently have physiologic adaptations to conserve moisture. Renal adaptations have allowed amphibians successfully to bridge the gap between aqueous and terrestrial habitats. The kidneys, skin, and, in many amphibian species, the urinary bladder play key roles in fluid homeostasis. Renal impairment may be responsible for the clinical manifestation of disease, morbidity, and mortality (Box 1).

Taxonomy

It is currently estimated that approximately 4000 known species of amphibians have adapted to a wide range of habitats but retain their dependency on water, particularly for reproduction. Many amphibian species are extensively used for research and teaching, with an increasing number finding their way into zoos and private collections.

The order Gymnophiona is composed of the caecilians, which number approximately 160 species and are poorly understood. They are generally nocturnal, legless, wormlike, burrowing amphibians from tropical areas worldwide and are rarely found in private collections or even zoologic institutions [1]. Two species occasionally seen in private collections and zoologic parks are the Mexican caecilian (*Dermophis mexicanus*) and the Varagua caecilian (*Gymnopis multiplicata*) [2].

The order Caudata accounts for approximately 350 species of vertebrates. This order includes the salamanders, newts, and amphiumas (Congo eels or eel newts). The terms "salamanders" and "newts" are often used interchangeably. The term "newt" is often associated with more aquatic

---

E-mail address: wetpetvet@aol.com

Box 1. Clinical signs of amphibian renal disease

- Lethargy
- Anorexia/Inappetence
- Weight loss/Emaciation
- Change in skin color or texture
- Coelomic distension ±ascites
- Change in urine output (anuria to polyuria)
- Death

---

species, whereas salamanders are traditionally creatures of damp and mossy woodlands [3]. Most members of the order Caudata are characterized by four legs and long tails, although there are exceptions. Several species fail to complete metamorphosis and retain external gill plumes throughout life (eg, axolotls) [4]. Salamanders such as sirens and amphiumas have reduced or absent rear limbs. Commonly kept salamanders include the Mexican axolotl (*Ambystoma mexicanum*), the tiger salamander (*Ambystoma tigrinum*), and the mud puppy (*Necturus* spp).

The last amphibian group is the order Anura, frogs and toads, which collectively number approximately 3400 species. They comprise the tail-less amphibians and possess strong hind jumping legs. Many species are popular in private collections, such as the leopard frog (*Rana pipiens*), the bullfrog (*Rana catesbeiana*), and the marine cane toad (*Bufo marinus*), with numerous other species commonly seen in private practice and zoologic institutions.

Renal anatomy

The basic excretory unit of the kidney in vertebrates, including fish, amphibians, reptiles, birds, and mammals, is the renal tubule or nephron. Its primary function is the maintenance of the desired water and solute concentration in the organism, that is, of a constant internal environment. Amphibian kidneys resemble those of freshwater teleost fish in that they lack the capability of concentration and can only produce hyposmotic urine. Only birds and mammals possess the ability to produce hyperosmotic urine [5]. Amphibians can decrease the rate of urine formation, and many can increase water resorption in the urinary bladder, thereby conserving fluids. Water resorption is controlled by the antidiuretic hormone, arginine vasotocin [6].

Amphibians possess separate and distinct renal systems for the larval and adult stages. The larval stage has a primitive aglomerular pronephric kidney located anterior to the later developing mesonephric kidney. The larval renal system consists of the paired pronephroi, which are organized in a segmented or metameric fashion along the dorsal aspect of the coelom. The pronephros consists of multiple nephrons, the number dependent on the species of amphibian. The primary function is to rid the body of nitrogenous waste in the form of ammonia and to maintain water homeostasis through the excretion of excess water. The pronephros filters coelomic fluid through a coelomostome or nephrostome. The coelomostome drains into a short tubule that serves as a filter but has no reabsorptive function. The pronephros also possesses primitive glomeruli that are outcroppings of the dorsal aorta, capable of limited blood filtration [7]. During metamorphosis the pronephros degenerates and is phagocytized, while the mesonephros begins to develop. Regression of the pronephroi and development of the mesonephroi are controlled by the thyroid hormones thriiodothyroxine and tetraiodothyroxine [8].

Most adult amphibians have different excretory needs from the larva. Metamorphic changes include renal adaptations that the aquatic-dependent larval forms will need to survive in a potentially part-aqueous, part-terrestrial existence. The kidneys are paired and located in the dorsal caudal coelomic cavity. The kidneys of adult terrestrial amphibians bear greater physiologic demands; they have evolved to excrete urea, and in rare instances uric acid, as the primary metabolic waste.

The kidneys of adult caecilians are fairly unchanged when compared with their larval stage, with the primary nitrogenous waste being ammonia. The caecilian kidney maintains its segmental shape, occupying the entire length of the coelomic cavity. The number of paired segments varies from 8 to 12, depending on the species, and they lack a distal tubule [7]. The kidneys function to filter both coelomic and vascular fluid. The kidneys empty through ureters into the neck of the bladder, which may be bilobate. The bladder then connects to the urodeum by a short urethra [9].

The salamander's anatomy pattern is consistent except for the presence of a distal tubule in all tailed amphibians except the amphiumas, whose mesonephroi resemble the kidneys of the adult caecilian. A greater number of nephrons are not connected to the coelomic cavity and lack a coelomostome, indicating a shift in importance from coelomic fluid filtration toward vascular filtration. The segmentation of the kidneys is reduced to five pairs in primitive salamanders and one to two pairs in terrestrial salamanders. The urinary bladder may be bilobate, bicornate, or cylindric. Terrestrial salamanders are able to excrete nitrogenous wastes as urea.

In anurans, the primary nitrogenous waste may be ammonia, urea, or uric acid. The more aquatic-dependent species excrete a higher concentration of ammonia. In general, the adult amphibian kidney still possesses two types of nephrons, coelomostomic nephrons and the more developed glomerular nephrons. The coelomostomic nephrons are located in a ventral position in the kidney and collect fluid directly from the coelomic cavity, with limited blood filtering function through a primitive glomerulus. The coelomostome has a ciliated neck portion, a proximal tubule, a second ciliated segment, and a distal tubule that connects to an archinephric duct. These primitive nephrons actively "sweep" coelomic fluid into the proximal tubule, where various electrolytes and glucose are reabsorbed. The second type of nephron, the glomerular nephron, lies dorsally in the kidney and is the primary blood filtering component of the amphibian kidney. Glucose, sodium, and chloride ions are actively reabsorbed in the proximal tubule. Additional salt is reabsorbed in the distal tubule along with passive resorption of water. In all, 99% of the total filtered ions are conserved. The glomerular filtration rate (GFR) of the amphibian kidney is high for vertebrates, ranging from 25 to 100 mL/kg/h, with a correspondingly high urine flow rate of 10 to 25 mL/kg/h [10]. Therefore, approximately half the primary filtrate is reabsorbed and half reaches the urinary bladder. Various physiologic parameters influence the GFR and urine flow rate, such as hydration and health status [11].

Renal physiology

Even though the body mass of most amphibians is composed of approximately 80% water, whereas most mammals are 65% water [12], amphibians do not drink water to replace fluid loss. Instead, they absorb fluids through the skin by osmosis [13]. Aqueous species face difficulty in limiting the uptake of water into the body, whereas terrestrial amphibians must conserve fluids and limit water evaporation and loss. Fluid homeostasis involves the balancing of absorption to loss and excretion. In most amphibians, the skin is a negligible barrier to water gain or loss. In drier conditions, transdermal evaporative fluid loss is high. In fresh-water habitats, water uptake is passive and under osmotic control [14]. Amphibian larval stages and all aqueous adult stages must excrete large amounts of dilute urine to compensate for fluid accumulation. Larval and aqueous adult amphibians are exclusively ammonotelic, with ammonia being highly water soluble but highly toxic. Animals that lack access to water environments will decrease their GFR, thereby accumulating ammonia in body tissues that may lead to azotemia and death.

With the exception of some tree frogs, most terrestrial amphibians are ureotelic (ie, they excrete urea as the primary nitrogenous waste product). At times of water deprivation, urea accumulates in the body's fluid compartments, but it is excreted rapidly on rehydration [15]. The leopard frog (*Rana pipiens*) will excrete approximately 80% of nitrogenous wastes as ammonia if the animal is properly hydrated [13]. Many terrestrial anurans have evolved metabolic adaptations to excrete urea, and even uric acid, as the primary nitrogenous waste product, thereby conserving fluids. *Bufo* spp are able to decrease their ammonia production to 5% and increase urea production, thereby sparing body water loss. Urea is less toxic than ammonia and may be stored in body tissues until water can be replenished. Some species of tree frogs (eg, African gray tree frog, *Chiromantis xerampelina*) have adapted to more arid habitats through the excretion of nitrogenous wastes as uric acid, as in reptiles and birds [13]. Many terrestrial species of amphibians are able to use the urinary bladder as a reservoir and actively reabsorb water to stave off dehydration [14].

Infectious causation

Bacterial diseases

Bacterial pathogens pose a high risk to animals that live immersed in a liquid environment where opportunistic bacteria are ubiquitous. Dermal lesions are most common, but penetration of the cutaneous layer can quickly lead to septicemia and potential nephritis. Reported causative agents of septicemia include *Pseudomonas fluorescens, Aeromonas hydrophila,* and several bacteria from the genera *Salmonella, Acinetobacter, Proteus,* and *Flavobacterium* [16–18]. *Chlamydia psittici* has been implicated in an outbreak of organ necrosis, including that of the kidneys, and acute bacterial septicemia in *Xenopus* spp [18].

Serotypes of *Leptospira interregans* have been detected in anurans serologically and by culture isolation, but no gross or histologic lesions have been noted [19].

Mycobacterial lesions have been recognized in several amphibian species, including the clawed frog (*Xenopus* sp) and Surinam toad (*Pipa pipa*) [15]. The acid-fast bacteria that affect amphibians (*Mycobacterium xenopei, M chelonae, M ranae, M ranicola, M glae*) [18] are ubiquitous in the environment and are considered a secondary pathogen. Immune-compromised individuals are most often affected because of primary disease, poor husbandry, or dermal injury. Poikilothermic strains of mycobacterium produce little or no exotoxin, and lesions do not caseate. Lesions are usually dermal, but chronic disease can proceed toward granulomatous lesions in any internal organ, including the kidneys [20]. Lesions develop over months, and death is due to organ dysfunction and failure.

Streptococcus spp were cultured at necropsy from an American bull frog (*Rana catesbeiana*) that succumbed to a necrotic hepatosplenitis and nephritis [15].

Viral diseases

Several viruses have been isolated from amphibians and associated with renal disease or damage, but documented reports are sparse. Tadpole edema virus is a Ranavirus type III that can affect various frogs (*Rana* spp) and toads (*Bufo* spp). The virus causes edema and dermal hemorrhage and can compromise the function of multiple organs, including the kidneys [15]. Frog virus 3 is a Ranavirus type I from the family Iridoviridae that has been documented to cause hemorrhage and necrosis in multiple organs, including the kidneys in leopard frogs. Bohle iridovirus causes viral hemorrhagic septicemia and nephritis and is fatal in various frog species. Luckè's herpesvirus, or ranid herpesvirus, has been identified as an initiating factor for renal carcinomas in northern leopard frogs and will be discussed in further detail later in this article, under neoplasia. The amphibian herpesviruses are phylogenetically distinct from the mammalian, avian, and reptilian herpesviruses, more closely resembling the herpesviruses that affect fish species. The ranid herpesvirus has been most closely related to the ictalurid herpesvirus 1, a virus that affects channel catfish [21].

Fungal diseases

Mucormycosis and zygomycosis are fungal infections caused by *Mucor* spp and *Rhizopus* spp, respectively. Mucormycosis seems to infect several species of anurans in Australia and is endemic in wild populations of cane toads (*B marinus*). Cutaneous nodules invade blood vessels, disseminate hematogenously to internal organs, including the kidneys, and form granulomas [22]. Chromomycosis has been attributed to the fungal genera *Cladosporium, Fonsecaea,* and *Phialophora* and affects multiple amphibian species. The disease is characterized by dermal nodules and disseminated granulomatous disease invading most internal organs, including the kidneys [15].

Parasitic diseases

Ciliated protozoa suspected to be *Entamoeba ranarum* was recovered from the kidney of the marine toad (*B marinus*) with subsequent suppurative tubular nephritis. The amoeba was described as being extracellular, 11 to 32 μm in diameter, and circular to ovoid in shape. The single nucleus possessed four nuclei, each 3 to 4 μm in diameter [23]. The ciliate *Trichodina urincola* has been recognized in the urinary bladder, skin, and gills of multiple anuran and caudate species with no pathologic lesions reported [19]. A coccidian parasite (*Isospora lieberkuehni*) has been rarely associated with renal disease and tubular nephritis in European anurans and fire-bellied toads (*Bombina variegata*) but has not proved to be a significant pathogen [24]. The coccidia are described as being slightly curved, approximately 7 μm long, and having an oocyte with 1 to 12 elongate merozoites in the cytoplasm [25].

A renal nematode was reported in a clawed frog (*Xenopus* sp) that presented with anorexia, color change, and "flaky skin." Subcutaneous nematodes (*Pseudocapillaroides xenopi*) were discovered, but histologic investigation found a nematode wrapped around the glomerulus in the Bowman's space. The renal nematode was not identified and is suspected to be an aberrant migratory nematode [26].

Monogenean trematodes, especially *Polystoma* spp, have been recovered from the intestinal tract, lungs, and urinary tracts of various species of anurans, with no significant lesions. Many genera of digenean trematodes (eg, *Alaria* spp, *Echinostoma* spp) use amphibians as intermediate hosts. Amphibians can serve as the final host for other trematodes, such as *Gorgodera amplicava*, which use the mesonephros for development and maturation and are common findings in the urinary bladder of anurans and salamanders of Europe, Africa, and North and South America [19]. Metacercarial cysts from *Clinostomum*, *Diplostomum*, and *Manidostomum* have induced granuloma formation in the kidneys and other internal organs. Flukes are noted as white nodules in the kidneys or bladder. Histologic changes usually present as encysted metacercariae or mesocercariae present in the renal interstitium, capsule, glomerular spaces, or tubules, with secondary changes of tubular dilation and necrosis. Clinical signs of trematode infestation include listlessness, anorexia, uremia, and potentially death due to ureteral or renal tubular obstruction.

A few myxozoan parasites have been found in multiple internal organs, including the kidneys of various amphibians. *Leptotheca ohlmacheri* is a common finding in the renal tubules of North American and European ranids, with no apparent pathologic lesions [27,28]. On death and histopathology of an Asian horned frog (*Megophrys nasuta*), a myxosporidean parasite (*Chlormyxum* sp) was associated with a suppurative interstitial nephritis, resulting in renal tubular dilation and necrosis [29]. A myxozoan parasite has been reported to cause polycystic renal disease in African hyperoliid frogs (*Hyperolius marmoratus*) and has been called "frog kidney enlargement disease." The new myxozoan species of *Hoferellus* has been implicated and has yet to be further identified [30].

Noninfectious causation

Dehydration

Dehydration and desiccation may affect all amphibians that are kept improperly. Toads and other terrestrial amphibians can return to a normal hydration status within 24 hours after access to water. Desert-adapted anurans can regain 30% of their body mass per hour during rehydration [31]. Urine production will return to normal when hydration status is improved.

Neoplasia

Renal carcinomas occur spontaneously in northern leopard frogs (*Rana pipiens*) and have been associated with Luckè's herpesvirus, also called ranid herpesvirus–1. The Luckè's tumor was first described in 1934, and earlier accounts date back to 1905 [31]. The neoplastic cells develop in the mesonephros and have the potential to metastasize to the liver, adipose, and urinary bladder [32]. Eggs, embryos, and larva exposed to the herpesvirus during spring breeding may develop the neoplasia. Leopard frogs are not susceptible to tumor development when first exposed as adults. Several features of the Luckè's herpesvirus are temperature dependent. Development of intranuclear inclusion bodies and virus formation and assembly occur in the "winter tumor" or during cooler weather conditions. Tumor growth, viral invasion, and metastasis occur during warmer periods or the "summer tumor" [19]. Clinical signs include coelomic distension, lethargy, and death due to renal failure or emaciation. Few animals show evidence of disease until the neoplasia is extensive [15].

Renal cell carcinomas were also reported in hybrids of the Japanese toad (*B japonicus*) and Chinese toad (*B raddei*) bred in a laboratory situation [33]. Electron microscopy showed no evidence of viral association.

Nephroblastomas have been reported in an African clawed frog (*X laevis*) and a fire-bellied newt (*Cynops pyrrhugaster*) [34,35]. The nephroblastoma is a true embryologic tumor of the mesonephric tissue. No tumors have been recorded in the pronephric tissues of any amphibian larval stage. Nephroblastomas have been experimentally induced in the Spanish ribbed newt (*Pleurodeles waltl*) by exposure during metamorphosis to the carcinogen N-methyl-N-nitrosouren [36].

The Registry of Tumors in Lower Vertebrates [37] has also received submission of a few renal tumors, including renal cell carcinomas in an African clawed frog, an ornate horned frog (*Ceratophry ornata*), and a mudpuppy (*Necturus maculosus*) (Fig. 1). Other neoplastic conditions from the amphibian urinary tract reported by the Registry include a urinary bladder lipoma in an African clawed frog, a myeloid leukemia in a marine toad, a paracloacal transitional cell carcinoma in a tiger salamander (*Ambystoma tigrinum*), and nodular lymphocytic hyperplasia in a mudpuppy.

Nutritional causes

Oxalate calculi were detected in the kidneys of leopard frog tadpoles that died at the time of metamorphosis. The tadpoles had been fed a diet high in chopped spinach and kale, which are high in oxalates [24]. A waxy frog (*Phyllomedusa sauvagii*) was reported to develop hydrocoelom, subcutaneous edema, and lethargy after being fed the silver queen, *Aslaonema ruebelinii*, an oxalate-producing plant. The diet was suspected to cause renal insufficiency, possibly owing to this frog's uricotelic nature and decreased urine production. Histologic evaluation of the kidneys revealed oxalate crystals [38].

The digits of a bullfrog (*Pixicephalus* spp) were reported to contain uric acid crystals (gout), which were thought to be the result of a high-protein diet [38]. However, the true cause was never determined.

Toxins

With their highly permeable dermis, the amphibians are sensitive to contaminants or toxins present in the water column that may impair renal function. For the most part, toxins that can produce illness in fish species should be considered toxic to amphibians. Factors that affect the toxicity of a chemical include temperature, pH, hardness, and alkalinity of the aqueous environment. Water parameters contribute to the patient's respiratory rate,

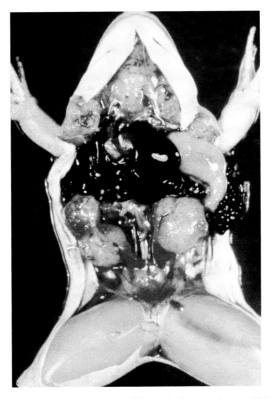

Fig. 1. Northern leopard frog (*Rana pipiens*) with renal adenocarcinoma. This image from Registry of Tumors in Lower Animals (RTLA) case 282 was obtained by using the services provided by the National Cancer Institute's RTLA, operated under contract by Experimental Pathology Laboratories, Inc. NO2-CB-27034. All rights reserved; with permission.

transdermal absorption, renal excretion, and detoxification mechanisms. Other considerations should include the health, size, and life stage of the exposed animal [39]. Definitive diagnosis should be based on history of exposure, exposure dose, and appearance of clinical signs consistent with the toxic agent.

Polyvinyl chloride (PVC) glue is used to cure or seal PVC pipe joints. When it is properly allowed to dry, no detectable levels are noted. Improper curing of the compound can cause it to dissolve in the water column, where it has been shown to be an irritant to the skin as well as cause renal failure [40]. PVC-associated toxicosis has been reported in poison arrow dart frogs exposed to a newly established habitat.

Heavy metals, such as copper, zinc, and lead, have been reported to damage the kidney function of multiple species and should be considered when evidence of renal toxicosis is present [24]. The most likely source of contamination with heavy metals is tainted water or copper-containing therapeutics. Water may be contaminated through copper, zinc, or lead piping that can leach into the water column. Clinical signs are consistent with renal and hepatic disease or failure (see Box 1). Diagnosis is difficult, but correlations may be drawn with clinical signs and high metal concentrations detected in the water habitat. Postmortem samples can be collected and submitted; they should include frozen liver, kidney, and muscle.

Diagnosis

Diagnostic procedures are often difficult in small species. Problems arise when one tries to correlate clinical pathology with disease. Hematology and biochemistry values are reported for many species, but there is tremendous variation due to sex, age, season, and state of hydration [15,19]. Diagnostic samples from healthy individuals in the same environment are important for comparison.

Blood collection in amphibians can be problematic because of animal handling, size of patient, and variable ability of laboratories to impart consistent results and interpretation. Phlebotomy is available through several vessels. The ventral abdominal vein lies superficially and is often difficult to access owing to its small size. The femoral and oral vessels may be used in larger species of amphibians, usually exceeding 100 g. Large anurans may be bled from cephalic veins with good restraint or anesthesia. Cardiocentesis or cardiac puncture is the preferred method for blood acquisition in most amphibians. The patient should be anesthetized and held in dorsal recumbency. A heparinized 25-gauge needle and syringe are inserted at a 45° angle distal to the xiphoid in a cranio-dorsal direction [40]. Veterinarians should choose a phlebotomy site depending on the patient's health status and size and the veterinarian's experience. In healthy reptiles, 1% of the body weight may be withdrawn for sampling (1 mL per 100 g of body weight), and this same rule may be applied safely to amphibians [41]. All locations for blood acquisition should be aseptically prepared to prevent the introduction of pathogens. As with reptiles, phosphorus may be used as an indicator of renal function, but normal values are lacking in most amphibian species. Calcium-to-phosphorus ratios should always be greater than one, with an inverted ratio suggestive of hypocalcemia, renal disease, or both. Most amphibians excrete at least some urea as a nitrogenous waste, but normal blood urea nitrogen values vary greatly depending on hydration status, seasonality, sex, age, and husbandry [42]. An elevated white blood cell count complemented by abnormal serum kidney parameters may be indicative of a renal infection.

Celiocentesis may be used to remove fluid from the coelomic cavity. Samples should be submitted for fluid analysis, including cytology, culture, and chemical analysis.

Urine samples may be readily collected from amphibians. Many amphibians will release a significant amount of urine when first handled. Cloacal stimulation with a small sterile rubber tube or moistened cotton-tipped applicator may also be used to collect urine. A sterile cup should be used to collect the sample. A wet mount should be inspected for cells and bacteria. A complete urinalysis provides important information, such as the presence of erythrocytes, inflammatory cells, casts, or bacteria [14].

Radiographic imaging of amphibians may be used to examine the skeletal, respiratory, and—to a limited degree—gastrointestinal systems. Details of other visceral organ systems (eg, kidneys) are poor because of the lack of abdominal adipose stores and soft tissue-gas interfaces. Calcification of renal tissue and the presence of cystic or renal calculi should be readily evident with standard radiographic techniques.

Renal biopsies may be used for diagnosis ante mortem and post mortem. Laparoscopic evaluation may be performed with a small-diameter rigid endoscope and a biopsy channel, with renal samplings submitted for culture and histology.

Therapeutics

Few pharmacokinetic studies have been reported for amphibian species. Variable metabolic rates, changes in physiologic activity, and different environmental conditions make standardization of dosages difficult. Any documented dosages should be used only as a guideline. Amphibians have a low metabolic rate but a high rate of fluid turnover, placing them between reptiles and mammals pharmacologically. Care should be taken to provide appropriate husbandry practices to maximize recovery (Box 2).

Methods of drug administration may be limited. Intravenous access is extremely difficult. Most amphibians are uncooperative during administration of oral medications. Forcing the mouth open can often result in a mandible

---

Box 2. Treatment protocol for amphibians with renal disease

A thorough history must be gathered, including husbandry practices, diet, acquisition and dispositions, recent health issues, and animal deaths.

Ideally, the housing should be inspected by the veterinarian with appropriate water quality parameters established.

Sick animals should be removed from a group situation, isolated, and housed in a quiet, clean environment suitable to the species.

Handling must be minimized to reduce stress.

Emergency care procedures must be expediently provided: celiocentesis, antibiotics, fluid therapy, and nutritional support as needed.

Appropriate diagnostic testing should be collected (eg, fecal evaluation, urinalysis, radiography, phlebotomy).

Table 1
Medications used in amphibians with suspected renal disease

Allopurinol	10 mg/kg PO q 24 h
Amphotericin B	1 mg/kg ICe q 24 h
Doxycycline	10–50 mg/kg PO q 24 h
Enrofloxacin	5–10 mg/kg IM, SQ, ICe, PO, TO q 24 h
Fenbendazole	100 mg/kg PO q 10–14 d
Itraconazole	2–10 mg/kg PO q 24 h
Ivermectin	0.2–0.4 mg/kg IM, PO q 10–14 d
Ketoconazole	10–20 mg/kg PO q 24 h
Levamisole	8–10 mg/kg ICe, TO, IM q 14 d
Metronidazole	50 mg/kg PO q 24 h
Oxytetracycline	50–100 mg/kg SQ, IM, PO q 48 h
Piperacillin	100 mg/kg SQ, IM q 24 h
Trimethoprim/sulfamethoxazole	15 mg/kg PO q 24 h

Abbreviations: ICe, intracoelomic; IM, intramuscular; PO, per os; SQ, subcutaneous; TO, topical.

fracture or torn skin around the face, but this maneuver may be facilitated with the use of a soft plastic card, speculum, or gentle traction. The skin on the dorsum is often thick and resistant to subcuticular injections, but the ventral skin is thinner and easier to penetrate. Often a ventral subcuticular injection enters the coelomic cavity to become an intracoelomic administration. Care must be taken to avoid perforation of internal organs. Intracoelomic injections are a viable mode of administration of various therapeutic drugs. Coelomic fluid is actively filtered by the kidneys and enters the general circulation, but clearance by excretion of aqueous medications could be rapid. Small patients have little muscle mass, but intramuscular injections may be given in the front limbs. Injections intended for systemic distribution should be avoided in the hind limbs owing to the presence of renal and hepatic portal systems. Fortunately, the skin of amphibians is extremely water soluble, allowing for transdermal application of aqueous agents by means of topical placement on the dorsal animal. Antimicrobial and antiparasitic therapy used to treat renal disease should be selected according to clinical signs and clinical conclusions. A good reference for therapeutics has been published by Carpenter [43] and Wright [44] (Table 1).

Acknowledgments

The author would like to thank Annette E. Henry, Survey Coordinator, Southwest Fisheries Science Center, La Jolla, California, for her assistance in obtaining reference material for this project.

References

[1] Mylniczenko ND. Caecilia (Gymniophona, Caecilia). In: Fowler M, editor. Zoo and wild animal medicine. 5th edition. Philadelphia: WB Saunders; 1999. p. 40–5.

[2] Wright K. Taxonomy of amphibians kept in captivity. In: Wright K, Whitaker BR, editors. Amphibian medicine and captive husbandry. Malabar (FL): Krieger Publishing; 2001. p. 3–6.

[3] Mattison C. The care of reptiles and amphibians in captivity. London: Bland Ford Press; 1991.

[4] Cranshaw G. Amphibian medicine. In: Bonagura J, editor. Kirk's current veterinary therapy XI: small animal practice. Philadelphia: WB Saunders; 1992. p. 1219–30.

[5] Schmidt-Nielsen K. Amphibians. In: Animal physiology. 5th edition. Cambridge (UK): Cambridge University Press; 1997. p. 355–73.

[6] Willmer P, Stone G, Johnston I. Environmental physiology of animals. Oxford (UK): Blackwell Science; 2000. p. 112–6.

[7] Wright K. Anatomy for the clinician. In: Wright K, Whitaker BR, editors. Amphibian medicine and captive husbandry. Malabar (FL): Krieger Publishing; 2001. p. 14–30.

[8] Duellman WE, Trueb L. Biology of amphibians. Baltimore (MD): Johns Hopkins University Press; 1994.

[9] Redrobe S, Wilkinson RJ. Reptile and amphibian anatomy and imaging. In: Meredith A, Redrobe S, editors. BSAVA manual of exotic pets. 4th edition. Gloucester (UK): British Small Animal Veterinary Association; 2002. p. 193–207.

[10] Withers C. Comparative animal physiology. Fort Worth (TX): Saunders College Publishing; 1992.

[11] Moberg N, Jespersen A, Wilkerson M. Morphology of the kidney in the West African caecilian, *Geotrypetes seraphini* (Amphibia, Gymnophiona, Caeciliidae). J Morphol 2004; 262(2):583–607.

[12] Schmidt-Nielsen K. Amphibians. In: Animal physiology. 2nd edition. Englewood Cliffs (NJ): Prentice-Hall; 1964. p. 37–45.

[13] Mattison C. Physiology. In: Frogs and toads of the world. London: Octopus Publishing; 1998. p. 16–28.

[14] Wright K. Applied physiology. In: Wright K, Whitaker BR, editors. Amphibian medicine and captive husbandry. Malabar (FL): Krieger Publishing; 2001. p. 31–4.

[15] Cranshaw G. Amphibian medicine. In: Fowler M, editor. Zoo and wild animal medicine: current therapy 3. Philadelphia: WB Saunders; 1993. p. 131–9.

[16] Emerson H, Norris C. "Red-leg, " an infectious disease of frogs. J Exp Med 1905;7:32–58.

[17] Urbain A. La paratyphose des grenouilles (*Rana esculenta*). J Soc Biol 1944;183:458–549.

[18] Temple R, Fowler M. Amphibians. In: Fowler M, editor. Zoo and wild animal medicine. Philadelphia: WB Saunders; 1978. p. 79–88.

[19] Green DE. Pathology of amphibia. In: Wright K, Whitaker BR, editors. Amphibian medicine and captive husbandry. Malabar (FL): Krieger Publishing; 2001. p. 401–85.

[20] Reichenbach-Klinke H, Elkin E. Bacterial diseases. In: Diseases of amphibians. New York: Academic Press; 1965. p. 221–46.

[21] Johnson AJ, Wellehan JFX. Amphibian virology. Vet Clin North Am Exot Anim Pract 2005;8:53–65.

[22] Parée JA. Fungal diseases of amphibians. Vet Clin North Am Exot Anim Pract 2003;6: 315–26.

[23] Valentine BA, Stoskopf MK. Amebiasis in a tropical toad. J Am Vet Med Assoc 1984;185: 1418–9.

[24] Cranshaw G. Anurans (Anura, Salienta): frogs, toads. In: Fowler M, editor. Zoo and wild animal medicine. 5th edition. Philadelphia: WB Saunders; 1999. p. 20–33.

[25] Levine ND, Nye RR. A survey of blood and other tissue parasites of leopard frogs, *Rana pipiens*, in the United States. J Wildl Dis 1977;13:17–33.

[26] Brayton C. Wasting disease associated with cutaneous and renal nematodes in commercially obtained *Xenopus laevis*. Ann N Y Acad Sci 1992;653:197–201.

[27] Kudo RR. On the protozoa parasitic in frogs. Trans Am Microsc Soc 1922;41:59–76.

[28] McKinnell RG. Incidence and histology of renal tumors of leopard frogs from north central states. Ann N Y Acad Sci 1965;126:85–98.

[29] Duncan AE, Garner MM, Bartholomew JL, et al. Renal myxosporidiasis in Asian horned frogs (*Megophrys nasuta*). J Zoo Wildl Med 2004;35(3):381–6.

[30] Mutschmann F. Pathological changes in African hyperoliid frogs due to a myxosporidian infection with a new species of *Hoferellus* (Myxozoa). Dis Aquat Organ 2004;60(3):215–22.

[31] Stacy BA, Parker JM. Amphibian oncology. Vet Clin North Am Exot Anim Pract 2004;7: 673–95.

[32] McKinnell RG, Cunningham WP. Herpesviruses in metastatic Luckè renal adenocarcinoma. Differentiation 1982;22(1):41–6.

[33] Masahito P, Shioka M, Kondo Y, et al. Polycystic kidney and renal cell carcinoma in Japanese and Chinese toad hybrids. Int J Cancer 2003;103(1):1–4.

[34] Meyer-Rochow VB, Asashima M, Moro SD. Nephroblastoma in a clawed frog *Xenopus laevis*. J Exp Anim Sci 1991;34(5–6):225–6.

[35] Zwart P. A nephroblastoma in a fire-bellied newt, *Cynops pyrrhugaster*. Cancer Res 1970; 30(11):2691–4.

[36] Green DE, Harshbarger JC. Spontaneous neoplasia in amphibian. In: Wright K, Whitaker BR, editors. Amphibian medicine and captive husbandry. Malabar (FL): Krieger Publishing; 2001. p. 333–400.

[37] Registry of Tumors in Lower Vertebrates. Available at: http://www.pathology-registry.com.

[38] Wright K, Whitaker BR. Nutritional disorders. In: Wright K, Whitaker BR, editors. Amphibian medicine and captive husbandry. Malabar (FL): Krieger Publishing; 2001. p. 73–84.

[39] Plumb JA. Toxicology and pharmacology of temperate freshwater fish. In: Stoskopf M, editor. Fish medicine. Philadelphia: WB Saunders; 1993. p. 311–22.

[40] Cooper JE. Urodela (Caudata, Urodela): salamanders, sirens. In: Fowler M, editor. Zoo and wild animal medicine. 5th edition. Philadelphia: WB Saunders; 1999. p. 33–40.

[41] Willette-Frahm M. Blood collection techniques in amphibians and reptiles. In: Bonagura J, editor. Kirk's current veterinary therapy XII: small animal practice. Philadelphia: WB Saunders; 1995. p. 1344–8.

[42] Hoegeman S. Diagnostic sampling of amphibians. Vet Clin North Am Exot Anim Pract 1999;3:731–9.

[43] Carpenter JW. Exotic animal formulary. 3rd edition. St. Louis (MO): Elsevier; 2005.

[44] Wright KM. Pharmacotherapeutics. In: Wright K, Whitaker BR, editors. Amphibian medicine and captive husbandry. Malabar (FL): Krieger Publishing; 2001. p. 309–30.

ELSEVIER
SAUNDERS

Vet Clin Exot Anim 9 (2006) 189–203

VETERINARY
CLINICS
Exotic Animal Practice

Index

Note: Page numbers of article titles are in **boldface** type.

A

Abdominal veins, in reptiles, anatomy of, 8

Acid-base homeostasis, as renal function, coelomic anatomy for, 1
in comparative species, 13–16. See also *specific species.*

Acute renal failure, in ferrets, 34–35
in mammals, 70, 78
treatment of, 81

Acute tubulonephrosis, in reptiles, 136

Adenovirus, renal disease caused by, in avians, 99

Adrenal glands, lack of, in fish, 19
renal disease associated with, in mammals, 79–80

Agenesis, of kidney, in rabbits, 49
in reptiles, 131

Albendazole, for encephalitozoonosis, in rabbits, 93–94

Aldosterone, renal regulation of, in invertebrates, 16

Aleutian disease (AD), in ferrets, 33–34, 91–92

Allopurinol, for renal disease, in amphibians, 186
in avians, 119–120
in reptiles, 172

Aminoglycosides, renal disease caused by, in avians, 111

Ammonia, renal processing of, physiology of, 14–16. See also *specific species.*
uricotely mechanism, 22–23

Amnion, in reptiles, 130

Amphibians, renal disease in, **175–188**
clinical signs of, 175–176
diagnosis of, 184–185
infectious causation of, 179–181

noninfectious causation of, 181–184
normal anatomy and physiology versus, 176–179
therapeutics for, 185–186
treatment protocol for, 185
renal system in, anatomy of, 5–6, 176–178
physiology of, 20–21, 178–179
taxonomy overview of, 175–176

Amyloidosis, renal disease caused by, in avians, 100–101
in hamsters, 59–61
in mammals, 90
in mice, 58–59
in reptiles, 141–142

Anabolic hormones, renal disease and, in reptiles, 172–173

Analgesics, for renal disease, in avians, 122

Anemia, with renal disease, in avians, 119
in mammals, 74, 78

Angiotensins, renal physiology of, in amphibians, 20
in birds, 23
in fish, 18–19
in mammals, 25
in vertebrates, 17

Antibiotics, for renal disease, in amphibians, 186
in avians, 119–121
nephrotoxicity precautions, 119, 122
renal disease caused by, in avians, 111

Antibody titers, for encephalitozoonosis diagnosis, in rabbits, 92–94

Antidiuretic hormone, renal regulation of, in invertebrates, 16
in mammals, 25–26

Antimicrobials, for encephalitozoonosis, in rabbits, 93–94
for renal disease, in amphibians, 186

doi:10.1016/S1094-9194(05)00082-4

Changing Your Address?

Make sure your subscription changes too! When you notify us of your new address, you can help make our job easier by including an exact copy of your Clinics label number with your old address (see illustration below.) This number identifies you to our computer system and will speed the processing of your address change. Please be sure this label number accompanies your old address and your corrected address—you can send an old Clinics label with your number on it or just copy it exactly and send it to the address listed below.

We appreciate your help in our attempt to give you continuous coverage. Thank you.

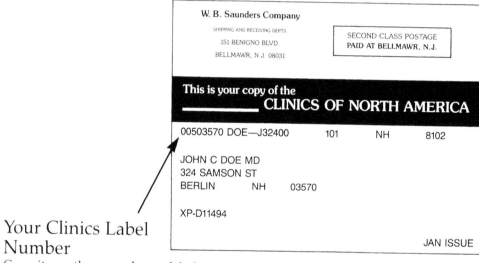

W. B. Saunders Company

SHIPPING AND RECEIVING DEPTS
151 BENIGNO BLVD.
BELLMAWR, N.J. 08031

SECOND CLASS POSTAGE
PAID AT BELLMAWR, N.J.

This is your copy of the

_____ CLINICS OF NORTH AMERICA

00503570 DOE—J32400   101   NH   8102

JOHN C DOE MD
324 SAMSON ST
BERLIN   NH   03570

XP-D11494

JAN ISSUE

Your Clinics Label Number

Copy it exactly or send your label along with your address to:
W.B. Saunders Company, Customer Service
Orlando, FL 32887-4800
Call Toll Free 1-800-654-2452

Please allow four to six weeks for delivery of new subscriptions and for processing address changes.